Svante Horsch · Kiriakos Ktenidis
Editors

CURRENT ASPECTS
IN VASCULAR SURGERY

Perioperative Monitoring in Carotid Surgery

Methods, Limits,
and Results

Long-term Results
in Carotid Surgery

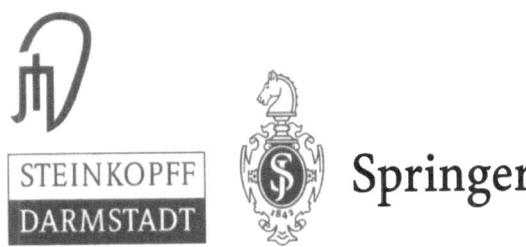

STEINKOPFF
DARMSTADT

Springer

Editors' addresses:

Prof. Dr. Svante Horsch
Dr. Kiriakos Ktenidis
Krankenhaus Porz am Rhein
Akademisches Lehrkrankenhaus der
Universität zu Köln
Klinik für Allgemeinchirurgie –
Gefäßchirurgie und Traumatologie
Urbacher Weg 19
51149 Köln

Die Deutsche Bibliothek – CIP-Einheitsaufnahme

Perioperative monitoring in carotid surgery : methods, limits and
results ; long-term results in carotid surgery / Svante Horsch ;
Kiriakos Ktenidis ed. – Darmstadt : Steinkopff ; Berlin ; Heidelberg ;
New York ; London ; Paris ; Tokyo ; Hong Kong ; Barcelona ;
Budapest : Springer, 1998
    (Current aspects in vascular surgery)

© Springer-Verlag Berlin Heidelberg 1998
 Originally published by Dr. Dietrich Steinkopff Verlag GmbH & Co. KG, Darmstadt
Softcover reprint of the hardcover 1st edition 1998
Medical Editor: Beate Rühlemann – English Editor: James C. Willis – Production: Heinz J. Schäfer
Cover Design: Erich Kirchner, Heidelberg

ISBN 978-3-642-95992-9   ISBN 978-3-642-95990-5 (eBook)
DOI 10.1007/978-3-642-95990-5

Preface

The efficiency of carotid surgery on an asymptomatic carotid artery stenosis and its superiority to conservative treatment was clearly demonstrated in the ACAS study. The stroke risk over a five year follow-up period could be reduced by 55 % and the combined stroke and mortality rate was shown to be a mere 2.3 %. The efficacy of surgical treatment in also reducing stroke rates in the case of a symptomatic carotid stenosis was proven in the NASCET and ECTS prospective randomized studies. Of extreme importance in these procedures is, however, precise quality control and quality assessment. This is presently a topic of tremendous interest in reconstructive vascular surgery and is constantly being discussed in specialist circles and beyond. Documentation and the possibility of accurate reconstruction of the intraoperative situation are in high demand.

Perioperative monitoring of neurological function, particularly the monitoring during carotid surgery, are the aspects underlying constant revision and reassessment to ensure quality control and assurance of a negligeable mortality and morbidity rate.

The aim of this book is to discuss the presently available perioperative control methods, examinations, and quality assessments, and the critical consideration of these.

We would like to express our thanks to all authors who helped achieve the sense and aim of this book.

A special word of thanks to Dr. Kerstin Simons (assistant surgeon) for assisting in the editing of the numerous presentations in this book. Particularly we thank Dr. Simons for the editing work in putting to paper the 'Consensus Conference on Perioperative Monitoring', which was documented on tape during the congress.

Also a sincere thank you to the publishers, Dr. Dietrich Steinkopff Verlag, for their support and assistance in making the completion of this book successful.

Cologne, April 1998   The Editors

Contents

Part I   Perioperative protection

Part II   Cerebral monitoring methods

Part III   Intraoperative control methods

Part IV   Intraoperative ICBP, EEG, and SEP monitoring

Part V   Intraoperative Transcranial Doppler sonography and oxymetry

Part VI   Short- and long-term results after carotid surgery

Part VII   Short- and long-term results after carotid surgery

Perioperative protection during carotid surgery on the part of the vascular surgeon

J. R. Allenberg

Department of Vascular Surgery, University of Heidelberg

It is naturally as important to the surgeon as it is to the anaesthetist or the neurologist that accurate intraoperative monitoring is conducted during carotid surgery. It goes without saying that the responsible surgeon is committed to applying a monitoring device that guarantees the highest available intraoperative safety.

The safety of carotid surgery does, however, not only commence intraoperatively, but already starts with the referring neurologist, who is required to select the patients who would benefit from surgery. An increased tendency among neurologists to opt for the more agressive, but significantly more effective surgical form of therapy is being noticed thanks to studies such as the NASCET and ECST. Patients are presently being referred, which would previously never have been subjected to a surgical consultation.

The preoperative neurological status is one of the vital factors influencing the postoperative success rate. This could be rephrased as "the healthier the patient, the better the results", but isn't it rather our duty to assist those who suffer from their carotid stenosis, and attempt to increase their quality of life? The aspect of an acute stroke following surgical intervention makes invasive therapies highly questionable. The collateral circulation is naturally of major influence in carotid clamping as are the patient's inherent risk factors, especially considering that half of all complications can be traced back to cardiac malfunction. To the surgeon, shunt insertion, various forms of cerebral monitoring (TCD, ICPB, SEP, EEG), as well as the control procedures (angioscopy and angiography) are of major importance. These procedures will be introduced individually in more detail later. A further important form of monitoring, which still requires mentioning, is intraoperative local or regional anaesthesia, which in my opinion is of particularly high value if used in combination with transcranial dopplersonography, even though it is not applied in the University of Heidelberg.

Using the example of an intraoperative angiography, the importance of monitoring and control techniques is demonstrated. In a prospective study, the value of angiography in 374 patients receiving carotid surgery was analyzed. Generally, the eversion-thrombendarterectomy technique was applied. The conventional method of a carotid patchplasty or prosthetic implantation was solely applied to carotid restenoses or carotid artery aneurysms. In 330 cases an intraoperative angiography was successfully completed. Apart from diagnosing pre-existing lesions, surgical problems were diagnosed and could be corrected: 11 patients showed evidence of a distal intimal step after endarterectomy, which required correction, and 2 patients exhibited a partial thrombosis. In two further cases, an occlusion had occurred, and another two demonstrated a stenosis caused by the suture. In six cases, occlusions of intracranial side branches were noted, although it has to be pointed out that four of these were preexisting in stroke-in-evolution-patients and only the remaining two could be ascribed to the surgical intervention. A successful lysis with 700.000 – 1.000.000 IU Urokinase was applied to these side branch occlusions. The overall morbidity and mortality rate of the presented patients was 1.9 %, despite 50 of these falling into the stage III patient group with an otherwise bleak prognosis.

Using the intra-operative on-table angiography, an instantaneous quality control of the reconstruction is available and documented. The angiography visibly presents technical faults immediately and makes a prompt correction possible.

This accurate form of representation of the intracranial branch-vessel situation makes it possible to pick up and effectively treat, by means of intraoperative lysis, the occlusions which may have developed during surgery or those already present in a stage III patient. Angiography in this form must also not be underestimated in its value in training a vascular surgeon, where the sudden appearance of an intimal flap after what was considered to be a flawless surgical procedure should be accompanied by the 'oh boy' experience.

In conclusion we consider an intraoperative quality control of our manual skill while performing a procedure for the benefit of a patient's rather vital organ, the brain, of major importance.

References

available from the author

Author's address:
J. R. Allenberg, MD
Section of Vascular Surgery
University of Heidelberg
Im Neuenheimer Feld 110
69120 Heidelberg, Germany

Perioperative protective procedures in carotid endarterectomy on the part of the anaesthesiologist

M. Abel, J. F. Meier

Department of Anaesthesiology and Pain Therapy, Krankenhaus Porz am Rhein, University of Cologne Teaching Hospital, Cologne

In dealing with patients for carotid surgery, the following considerations are particularly important:
▶ risk factors, pre-existing diseases and preoperative anxiolysis
▶ intraoperative analgesia and immobility of operation site
▶ adequate monitoring to prevent ischaemia
▶ optimum cerebral blood-flow.

Risk factors, pre-existing diseases and preoperative anxiolysis

Patients with cerebrovascular disease often present with characteristic risk factors and complex morbidity (3). The individual situation is assessed and quantified through knowledge of the patient's history, previous findings and specific preoperative diagnosis. In conclusion, the specific preoperative risk is classified according to ASA standards, any additionally necessary prior treatment resulting is indicated, and the suitable anaesthetic procedure decided on (3, 6, 10).

Preoperative anxiety and restlessness cause an increase in heart rate, peripheral vascular resistance, systemic blood pressure and myocardial oxygen consumption. The pre-anaesthetic visit, anxiolytic medication and the continuation of antihypertensive and cardiac medication all serve to prevent intra- and postoperative cardiocirculatory dysfunction and consecutive neurological damage. Heavy sedation should be avoided because of the risk of respiratory and circulatory depression. The preoperative preparation minimizes the perioperative risk for the patient (3, 4, 6, 10).

Adequate anaesthetic procedures

General, regional and combined anaesthetic procedures are used for carotid surgery, but are judged controversely as to their suitability.

Quite early, carotis surgery was performed on patients only with cervical ganglion block for analgesia. Arguments in favour of this procedure are the minimum exposure to anaesthetics and the maintained vigilance of the patient, which can be made use of in the sense of "direct neuromonitoring". Reports of recent anaesthesiological experience show problems with stress avoidance and blood pressure regulation during regional anaesthesia (1, 2, 3, 8, 9, 13). In fact, only general anaesthesia allows "intraoperative discomfort" to be reliably eliminated and guarantees the complete motor block of the operation site. A basic advantage of general anaesthesia over regional anaesthesia lies in the fact that both cerebral blood flow (CBF) and cerebral oxygen consumption (CMRO2) can be actively influenced (3, 5, 8). With a choice of different methods of ventilation, the combination of intravenous and volatile anaesthetics and the use of various substances to control blood pressure, the anaesthetist has many different possibilities to optimize the cerebral and cardiac ratios of oxygen delivery and requirement (3, 7, 9, 10). In the event of intraoperative complications, under general anaesthetic therapeutic hypertension or controlled hypothermia can be quickly induced, or cerebral metabolism suppressed with barbiturates (10).

In a risk versus benefit analysis in their own clinic, the authors have come out in favour of total intravenous anaesthesia (TIVA) with continuous application of propofol and alfentanil or fentanyl in bolus form. Study data show that cerebral oxygen uptake under anaesthesia with propofol was 36 % less than when awake. The cerebral venous oxygen saturation dropped from 64 % to 55 %, from which can be concluded that oxygen extraction from the blood is increased. Cerebral blood vessel reaction to CO_2 is maintained under propofol. Similar to thiopental and etomidate, propofol reduces cerebral oxygen consumption and is therefore considered to protect the brain (12). Patients who undergo anaesthesia with propofol, fentanyl/alfentanil and titrated doses of muscle relaxants can be extubated and neurologically assessed immediately following surgery. Normally they return to the general surgical ward after 6 – 8 h intensive care.

Monitoring for ischaemia prevention

Basic monitoring in carotid surgery should include continuous invasive measurement of blood pressure, pulse oximetry and capnometry. Ischaemia during carotid clamping can be clearly identified in an uncomplicated manner by registering somatosensory evoked potentials (SEP), which is just as reliable as neurological monitoring of the awake patient (5). SEP monitoring can therefore be routinely recommended for carotid surgery. In the authors' clinic, transcranial Doppler ultrasound is used to monitor cerebral bloodflow and for early detection of clamping ischaemia. Although this can also be used to detect precursory neurological deficits, the method fails in approximately half of all patients with preexisting insufficient collateral circulation (3, 5).

Available literature describes EEG methods as useful but not obligatory due to their restricted sensitivity and specificity (5, 14).

The continuous measurement of oxygen saturation in the jugular vein is regarded as a reliable indicator of the ratio of total cerebral blood supply and total cerebral oxygen consumption. However, regional changes in cerebral blood flow cannot always be documented with this method.

Up to now, there is no reliable indication that a certain monitoring technique guarantees optimum patient outcome (3).

Optimum cerebral bloodflow

Permissive hypercarbia, which is often used to improve cerebral bloodflow, can cause steal phenomena in patients with cerebrovascular insufficiency. For them, hypocarbia will therefore be more favourable, inducing so-called "inverse steal" with bloodflow redirected to ischaemic areas (3). For special-risk patients, the perioperative incidence of stroke can be reduced by the use of a shunt and selective bloodflow increase, e.g. with short-acting positive inotrope and vasopressor drugs (5, 11).

References

1. Becquemin JP, Paris E, Valverde A, Pluskwa F, Melliere D (1991) Carotid surgery. Is regional anesthesia always appropriate? J Cardiovasc Surg 32: 592
2. Breek JC, Peters N, Dewitte R, Bleyn J (1994) Carotid surgery under locoregional anaesthesia. Description of technique and results of our first 100 consecutive operations. Acta Chir Belg 94: 274
3. Clark JN, Stanley TH (1990) Anesthesia for Vascular Surgery. In: Miller RD (Ed) Anesthesia, 2nd edit. Churchill Livingstone, New York Edinburgh London Melbourne Tokyo
4. Cox C, Bannister J (1994) Anaesthesia for carotid artery surgery. Br J Anaesth 72: 252
5. Dinkel M (1995) Neuromonitoring in der Karotischirurgie. Anaesthesist 44/S2, 213
6. Eyrich K (1979) Sorgfalt bei der Prämedikation und Wahl des Anästhesieverfahrens. Anaesth Intensivmed 20: 39
7. Michenfelder JD, Sundt TM, Fode N et al. (1987) Isoflurane when compared to enflurane and halothane decreases the frequency of cerebral ischaemia during carotid endarterectomy. Anesthesiology 67: 336
8. Moreau P, Bonnaure E (1993) Reflexions a propos de la protection cerebrale dans la chirurgie carotidienne. Ann Chir 47: 742
9. Pluskwa F, Bonnet F, Saada M, Macquin-Mavier I, Becquemin JP, Catoire P (1991) Effects of clonidine on variation of arterial blood pressure and heart rate during carotid artery surgery. J Cardiothor Vasc Anaesth 5: 431
10. Roizen MF (1993) Role of the anesthesiologist in vascular procedures. J Cardiothor Vasc Surg 7: 257
11. Smith JS, Roizen MF, Cahalan MK et al. (1988) Does anesthetic technique make a difference? Augmentation of systolic blood pressure during carotid endarterectomy: Effects of phenylephrine versus light anesthesia and of isoflurane versus halothane on the incidence of myocardial ischemia. Anesthesiology 69: 846
12. Stephan H, Sonntag H, Schenk HD, Kohlhausen S (1987) Einfluß von Disoprivan (Propofol) auf die Durchblutung und den Sauerstoffverbrauch des Gehirns und die CO_2-Reaktivität des Hirnkreislaufs. Anaesthesist 36: 60
13. Tokolander R, Bergqvist D, Hulthen UL, Johannson A, Katzman PL (1990) Carotid artery surgery. Local versus general anaesthesia as related to sympathetic activity and cardiovascular effects. Eur J Vasc Surg 4: 265
14. Zickmann B, Knothe C, Boldt J, Hempelmann G (1992) Risikominderung in der Anästhesie – Einfluß des Monitorings. Anästh Intensivmed 33: 131

Author's address:
M. Abel, M.D.
Dept. of Anaesthesiology and Pain Therapy
Krankenhaus Porz am Rhein
University of Cologne Teaching Hospital
51145 Cologne, Germany

Perioperative monitoring of cerebral tissue oxygenation

M. A. Weigand, H. J. Bardenheuer

Department of Anesthesiology, University of Heidelberg, Heidelberg

Introduction

While clinical evaluation was one of the earliest approaches to judge cerebral function, the development of computer technology has made it possible to monitor cerebral perfusion and cerebral functions nearly on a real time basis. Today somatosensory evoked potential (SSEP) monitoring is the "gold standard" of cerebral evaluation during carotid artery surgery. Near infrared spectroscopy has been recently applied to measure cerebral hemodynamics noninvasively and continuously and may improve the quality of clinical treatment.

Physiology of cerebral blood flow

With a weight of approximately 1350 g the human brain represents about 2 % of total body weight. However, it receives 12–15 % of cardiac output, which reflects the high cerebral metabolic rate. At rest, cerebral blood flow is 40–60 ml/min/100 g of brain tissue and the brain consumes 2.9–3.5 ml/min/100 g oxygen. This is about 20 % of total body oxygen consumption. With 5.1 ml/min/100 g of brain blood flow is fourfold higher to the gray matter compared with white matter (14, 36).

While 60 % of cerebral oxygen consumption is used for electrophysiologic function such as depolarization – repolarization activity, the remaining 40 % is used to maintain cellular homeostasis (14). Since increases in cerebral oxygen requirements must be matched by proportional changes in cerebral blood flow, there is a local "coupling" between cerebral metabolic rate (CMR) and cerebral blood flow (CBF). The close "coupling" between regional cerebral blood flow and cellular metabolism is managed by local release of metabolic by-products. Adenosine, potassium and calcium ions seem to be the most important mediators which adjust cerebral vascular tone (32, 47). In addition to local metabolic regulation, cerebral vascular resistance in normal subjects is adjusted by myogenic regulation in the range between 50 and 150 mmHg (autoregulation). It is of clinical relevance that sympathetic nerve stimulation shifts the lower and upper end of the autoregulation plateau to the right (24). Therefore, moderate levels of hypotension can be associated with enhanced risk of inadequate cerebral perfusion under conditions of increased sympathetic activity.

Changes in $PaCO_2$ can directly increase cerebral blood flow (1 mmHg $PaCO_2$ increases CBF by 1–2 ml/min/100 g of brain tissue) (46). In contrast, arterial oxygen partial pressure (PaO_2) exerts only minimal changes of CBF over a wide range of 60 to 300 mmHg. A substantial rise, however, can be obtained, when PaO_2 falls below 60 mmHg (14).

Reflected by "slowing" of the EEG ischemic neuronal dysfunction occurs, when local cerebral blood flow falls to approximately 20 ml/min/100 g of brain tissue. Below a level of 12–15 ml/min/100 g of CBF cortical EEG becomes isoelectric, and delayed neuronal death occurs at a flow range between 6 and 12 ml/min/100 g (1, 4, 5, 49). When cerebral arteries are occluded, collateral blood flow is provided via circulus arteriosus Willisii as well as via distal branches of the internal and external carotid artery. Under these conditions there is a change in the direction of flow in the ophtalmic artery (8).

Monitoring of cerebral perfusion with electroencephalography (EEG)

At present there is no method available that provides fast, noninvasive and accurate monitoring of local as well as global cerebral blood flow in the intraoperative setting (17, 43). Although [133]Xenon, stable Xenon-enhanced computed tomography, positron emission tomography, single-photon emission computed tomography (SPECT) and the technique described by Kety and Schmidt (25) are generally available under clinical conditions, they can not be used for the acute and intraoperative measurement of flow changes. On the other hand, most procedures (which are described in this review) do not measure true flows but rather provide indices that can be related to flow changes.

Changes in EEG activity are the result of rhythmic excitation of cortical neurons. Since electrical activity is based on sufficient cerebral oxygenation and integrity of cellular membranes, the EEG can be taken to indirectly reflect disturbances in tissue oxygenation.

Basics of the EEG

The EEG signal contains four basic parameters: amplitude, frequency, time and characteristic patterns like "burst suppression" or "spikes and waves". In the awake patient with the eyes open, the physiologic basal frequency is termed β-range (> 13 Hz). After eye closure, the predominant frequency is the α-range between 8 to 13 Hz. θ- (4–7 Hz) and φ- (< 4 Hz) frequencies occur during sleep, cerebral abnormalities and anesthesia, respectively. The EEG is termed "depressed" when lower frequencies predominate (44). In contrast to bilateral ischemia, unilateral ischemic events are more easily detected, because the contralateral non ischemic brain hemisphere can serve as a control, such as during cardiac and carotid artery surgery.

Processed EEG

In clinical practice the analog signal of the standard EEG is digitalized and mathematically transformed (3). Although this procedure may lead to some loss of information of the standard EEG, the power spectral analysis by Fourier transformation converts irregular EEG waves to equivalent sine waves of known frequency and amplitude (31, 44).

Following transformation, the processed EEG can be displayed in a three- (compressed spectral array (CSA)) or a two-dimensional diagram (density spectral array (DSA)) and the following parameters can be used for monitoring of cerebral perfusion: absolute and relative band power as well as median and spectral edge frequency, respectively. In general, ischemia is detected by a reduction of the numbers of fast frequencies and an increase in the rate of slow frequencies.

Clinical application and limits of EEG monitoring

Under certain conditions of cardiac and carotid artery surgery EEG has been used for cerebral monitoring. In patients with carotidendarterectomy, however, Lam et al. (29) found that somatosensory evoked potentials (SSEP) were superior to EEG monitoring in the detection of focal cerebral ischemia. This result was confirmed by Langer et al. (30), who examined 68 patients with computer-aided electroencephalographic monitoring. The criteria for cerebral ischemia were the increase of slow frequencies and the decrease of fast frequencies by more than 50 %, respectively. In 9 % of the patients EEG monitoring was not possible at all. Five of 11 patients with pathological EEG showed no significant changes in SSEP and no neurological alterations postoperatively. Assuming a shunt was placed based on EEG changes, the shunt frequency would have been too high. Langer et al. (30) concluded that EEG monitoring during carotid artery surgery is not sensitive enough to distinguish between patients with and without adequate cerebral collateral circulation. Similar results were obtained during cardiac surgery, when no significant correlation was found between EEG changes and postoperative neuropsychological deficits in patients undergoing cardiopulmonary bypass (2).

Using EEG for monitoring of cerebral perfusion, one has to consider that anesthetic drugs, surgical factors and pathophysiologic factors can directly influence the EEG tracing. Subanesthetic doses of both intravenous and inhaled anesthetics produce an increase in frontal β-activity, whereas anesthetic doses evoke a slowing of EEG. In high concentrations some anesthetics cause a burst suppression pattern and even electrocortical silence. The application of opioids cannot produce an isoelectric EEG.

Hypothermia and pathophysiologic changes that occur with the institution of cardiopulmonary bypass may cause EEG changes that are comparable to those obtained with inadequate cerebral blood flow. Therefore, adequate cerebral monitoring using EEG may be difficult, if not impossible to be interpreted correctly during extracorporeal circulation (3, 11, 15, 17).

Evoked potential monitoring of cerebral perfusion

Intraoperative monitoring of evoked potentials has gained an increasing importance in the detection of functional integrity of sensoric pathways which are at risk during surgical procedures. Evoked potentials are electrophysiologic manifestations of the CNS response to external stimuli (11, 14). Depending on the mode of stimulation, auditory (AEP)-, brain stem auditory (BAEP)-, visual (VEP)- and somatosensory (SSEP)- evoked potentials can be differentiated. Because of the low amplitude of evoked potentials in the range of 0.1–20 µV, repetitive stimulation with averaging and amplification of the signals is necessary to distinguish evoked potentials from background activity (3, 26). For intraoperative monitoring of the central nervous system, short-latency SSEP are most commonly used, because SSEP are less influenced by anesthetics. Since motor evoked potentials are very sensitive to anesthetic factors, they are not suitable for intraoperative monitoring of the central nervous system (52). In anesthesia and critical care medicine, auditory evoked potentials have been mainly used during procedures involving the auditory pathway and posterior fossa (3). These potentials were used to either monitor depth of anesthesia (51), or to evaluate the prognosis of patients with severe head injury. For instance, intraoperative awareness was studied using midlatency auditory evoked potentials (45). Visual evoked potentials are no reliable parameters during surgery, because of the high incidence of both false-positive and false-negative results (3).

According to the site of stimulation, somatosensory potentials (SSEP) can be evoked by the stimulation of N. medianus or N. tibialis, respectively. While tibialis SSEP assess the functional integrity of the spinal cord, medianus SSEP have mainly been used to detect cerebral ischemia. In particular, medianus SSEP are very sensitive to changes in blood flow of the A. cerebri media. Furthermore, Craft et al. (9) found that the frontoparietal recording electrodes of the EEG are the most sensitive to detect cerebral ischemia during carotid artery surgery.

Somatosensory evoked potentials are sensitive to changes in blood pressure, body temperature, blood gas tensions, and hematocrit (21, 41). In contrast to the EEG, however, SSEP monitoring is applicable during moderate anesthesia, even at such plasma levels of barbiturates that cause isoelectricity in the EEG. On the other hand, when isoflurane is used at 1.5 MAC and at higher ranges, the electrical response upon SSEP stimulation disappears (13). As long as the concentration of volatile anesthetics is kept below 1 MAC, the ability to monitor cortical SSEP as a reliable parameter of cerebral perfusion is preserved (39, 40, 42). Even under high doses of opioids, SSEP monitoring is usually possible. While most anesthetics produce an increase in central conduction time and a decrease of SSEP amplitude, etomidate increases the amplitude (26, 27). On the other hand, hypothermia, nitrous oxide and hypotension decrease the SSEP amplitude (40). In summary, SSEP is less influenced by factors such as anesthesia or hypothermia than EEG. One major advantage of SSEP over EEG is the existence of easily interpretable and reliable criteria for cerebral ischemia.

Clinical importance of SSEP monitoring

In clinical studies intraoperative SSEP monitoring has been demonstrated to be an indicator of disturbances in cerebral tissue perfusion. For instance, Dinkel et al. (12) studied 753 patients undergoing carotidendarterectomy in which insufficient collateral blood flow (7 %) could be identified by complete loss of SSEP amplitude. Only five patients without an intraoperative complete loss of SSEP exhibited postoperative neurological deficits, which were related to thrombembolism. Three of 12 patients with SSEP loss, but without shunt placement showed no neurological deficits in contrast to 28 patients (out of 38) with shunt placement. Dinkel et al. (12) concluded that total loss of SSEP amplitude is a very sensitive and specific parameter to detect critical cerebral hypoperfusion during carotid artery surgery. Figure 1 illustrates the concept of selective shunting. After clamping of the carotid artery, the SSEP amplitude (N20/P25) progressively decreases. The complete loss of the SSEP amplitude during vessel occlusion is taken to be an absolute indication for shunt placement. After shunt placement, the SSEP amplitude continuously increases indicating sufficient recovery of neuronal function.

Although SSEP are taken as the "gold standard" to indicate inadequate cerebral perfusion, our own results demonstrate that the changes in SSEP exhibit a significant time delay after clamping in comparison to other indicators, such as regional cerebral oxygen saturation (NIRS) (Table 1). In addition, there is strong evidence that the changes in SSEP show a large interindividual variation and are not homogeneous during the clamping period. As is shown in Table 2, SSEP amplitude decreased in 23 patients from baseline value (100 %) to 80 % within 10 min after clamping. In 8 patients (26 %), however, there was actually an increase in SSEP amplitude by 45 % after acute occlusion of carotid artery.

Despite the fact that there is ongoing research concerning the sensitivity and specifity of medianus SSEPs, monitoring of somatosensory evoked potentials is a standard procedure

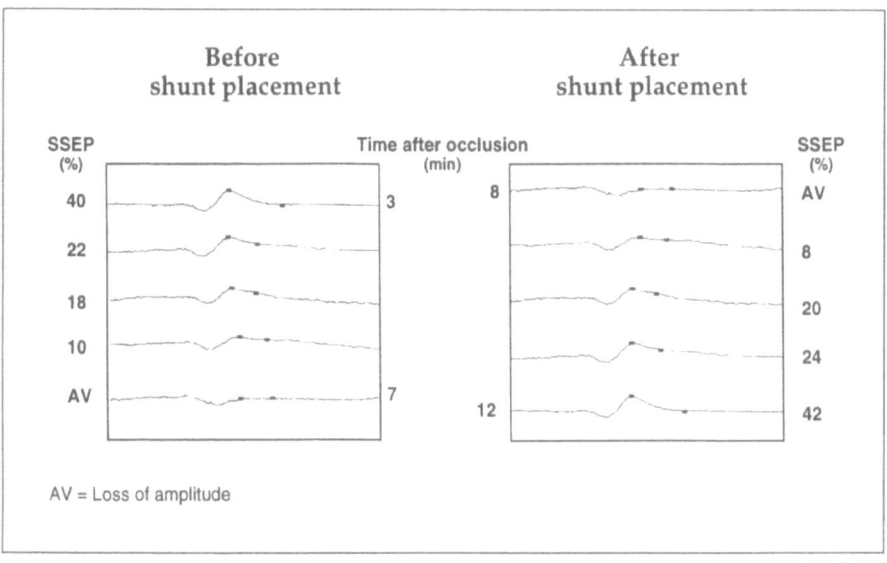

Fig. 1. Tracing of SSEP during carotid artery surgery. Total recovery of SSEP signal was reached after shunt placement.

Table 1. Time delay of maximal changes in SSEP and rSO_2 after carotid artery clamping

	SSEP	rSO_2	Difference ($SSEP - rSO_2$)
Time after carotid occlusion (min)	13.5 ± 3.7	4.5 ± 3.1	6.5 ± 3.2

Median ± 95 % CI

Table 2. Comparison of changes in SSEP and rSO_2 during carotid artery occlusion

Time after occlusion	SSEP (% of control)				rSO_2 (%)			
	1'	5'	10'	20'	1'	5'	10'	20'
group A (n = 23)	91 ± 9	84 ± 6	80 ± 7	85 ± 6	65 ± 1	64 ± 1	63 ± 1	65 ± 1
group B (n = 8)	103 ± 10	119 ± 15	142 ± 12	130 ± 12	66 ± 3	65 ± 4	65 ± 4	66 ± 3
A + B (n = 31)	94 ± 7	94 ± 7	98 ± 8	97 ± 7	65 ± 11	64 ± 2	64 ± 1	65 ± 1

Baseline values before carotid artery occlusion: SSEP = 100 %; rSO_2 = 70 ± 3 % (Mean ± SE)

during carotid artery surgery. It has to be remembered, however, that neuronal function parameters, such as EEG and evoked potentials, can only indirectly reflect the adequate cerebral oxygenation. From a functional point of view, both methods reflect "late parameters", because changes in SSEP are preceded by changes in cerebral oxygenation. Therefore, the current research is focused to more directly register quantitative changes in cerebral tissue oxygenation.

Near infrared spectroscopy (NIRS)

Near infrared spectroscopy was first introduced by Jobsis (23) and is a noninvasive method to monitor cerebral oxygenation. Similar to pulse oxymetry, near infrared spectroscopy uses attenuation of light by oxy- and deoxyhemoglobin to measure changes in blood oxygenation (16). Light in the visible spectrum ($\lambda = 400$–700 nm) has long been used to measure oxygen content of whole blood. However, visible light is not suited to measure tissue oxygen, because it penetrates tissue only by a few millimeters and is highly absorbed (16). In contrast, near infrared light in the spectral range ($\lambda = 700$–1000 nm) penetrates tissue up to 8 cm (16, 54) and is reflected by the chromophores oxyhemoglobin (HbO_2), deoxyhemoglobin (Hb) and cytochrome aa_3 (cyt aa_3 = cytochrome oxidase c) in brain tissue (34).

Oxyhemoglobin, deoxyhemoglobin and oxidized cytochrome aa$_3$

Changes of oxy- and deoxyhemoglobin can be used to estimate the oxygenation of cerebral hemoglobin, cerebral blood volume and cerebral perfusion (6, 28, 38). The redox potential of cytochrome aa_3 which is the final enzyme of the respiratory chain is of highest importance for oxidative metabolism. It has to be mentioned that more than 90 % of oxygen consumed by humans involve a reaction catalyzed by the cytochrome oxidase. In the final step of the respiratory chain, cytochrome oxidase donates electrons and protons to molecular oxygen to produce water, and becomes oxidized in this process. In the absence of oxygen, however, electron transfer cannot take place and, as a consequence, electrons accumulate on the heme and copper atoms of cytochrome aa_3 (6). There is a direct coupling of the redox state of cyt aa_3 to the quotient of phosphocreatine and anorganic phosphate (50). Sylvia et al. (48) demonstrated in the parietal cortex of rats that changes of the redox state of cyt aa_3 are closely followed by changes of phosphocreatine. Note that the reduction of cytochrome oxidase occurs before the decrease in phosphocreatine and adenosine triphosphate, respectively. In animal experiments, there was a close relationship between changes in cyt aa_3 and β-ATP, measured with near infrared spectroscopy and noninvasively analyzed by ^{31}P-NMRS, respectively (33). Tamura et al. (50) showed almost identical values for oxidized cytochrome aa_3 during perfusion with blood as well as during perfusion with fluorocarbon. This result supports the hypothesis that attenuation of light by cyt aa_3 can be distinguished from light absorption by hemoglobin.

Differences among near infrared spectroscopy

Infrared light is generated by laser diodes, the light of which is captured in glass fiberoptic strands that form a bundle carrying light to an optode on the patients head. An identical fiberoptic system which is approximately 4–8 cm apart from the first optode collects the light photons and conducts them back to a detector. Different near infrared devices vary in their sources of monochromatic light, the number of wavelengths used, and the mathematical algorithm to calculate HbO_2, Hb, Cyt aa_3 or regional cerebral oxygen saturation (rSO_2), respectively (6). For transillumination, which is only possible in newborns, the light source and light receiver are placed on opposite sites of the head. In older children or adults, the light source and receiver are placed closer together at a distance of about 4–7 cm and a wedge of brain tissue is monitored. While transillumination allows global measurement of cerebral oxygenation, only regional oxygenation can be monitored in adults (34, 54). The spacing of the light source and sensors determines the field sampled (34). Near infrared monitors currently in use are the Niro 500 (Hamamatsu), the Cerebral Oxymeter Invos 3100A (Somanetics) and the Cerebral RedOX Research Monitor model 2001 (Criticon). Differences of these monitors are not discussed.

Clinical application of near infrared spectroscopy

Figure 2 shows the tracing of regional cerebral oxygen saturation and the amplitude of somatosensory evoked potentials during carotid artery surgery. Because of the total loss of SSEP amplitude, a shunt was intraoperatively placed. This example can be used to discuss advantages and disadvantages of both NIRS and SSEP monitoring:

There is a quick decrease and increase of rSO_2 after occlusion and reperfusion of carotid artery. During reperfusion, the transient increase of rSO_2 above baseline values reflect the changes in flow during reactive hyperemia (29). Changes of rSO_2 significantly precede alterations of SSEP. While total loss of SSEP amplitude is considered to be a clear signal of inadequate collateral blood flow, rSO_2 does not furthermore fall to indicate critical cerebral hypoperfusion in this particular example.

While rSO_2 totally recovered at the end of the observation period, SSEP values remained below baseline values. This prolonged recovery of neuronal function is likely to

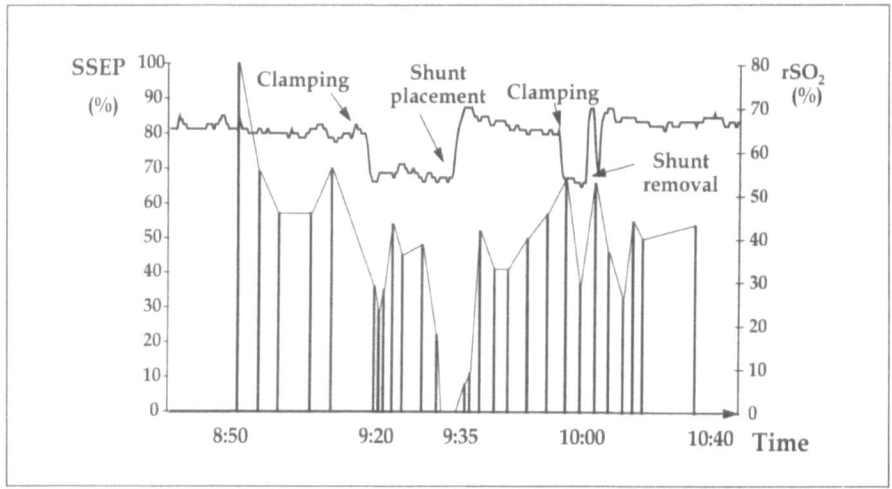

Fig. 2. Changes of regional cerebral oxygen saturation (rSO$_2$) and SSEP before and after shunt placement in a patient with inadequate collateral blood flow.

signal reperfusion damage. Intraoperative monitoring of cerebral perfusion should give a clear indication when a shunt has to be placed. Today SSEP monitoring is the standard in carotid artery surgery. In addition, the total loss of SSEP amplitude is the indication for shunt placement. On the other hand, a critical value for rSO$_2$ is not yet defined. In consideration of our own data, the relative decrease of rSO$_2$ seems to be a better parameter for the detection of critical cerebral hypoperfusion than the absolute value of rSO$_2$.

In addition, rSO$_2$ is a very early indicator of cerebral ischemia (see Table 1). This finding is confirmed by Williams et al. (53) who found parallel and rapid changes of rSO$_2$, blood flow velocity and jugular venous oxygen saturation during carotid artery occlusion.

Limits of near infrared spectroscopy

The results of two recent studies suggest that regional cerebral oxygen saturation, measured with the Somanetics device, does not determine intracerebral, but only extracerebral oxygen saturation. Harris et al. (22) studied rSO$_2$ (Invos, Somanetics) and blood velocity of middle cerebral artery (vMCA) in 10 patients requiring controlled ventilation during minor surgery. The Invos probe was placed on the forehead with optodes 1.0 and 2.7 cm apart from each other. When FECO$_2$ of 3 kPa was reached by hyperventilation, carbon dioxide was additionally applied to stepwise increase FECO$_2$ up to 6.0 kPa by 0.2 kPa. Under these conditions, vMCA increased by more than 100 % which was associated with only minor increases in rSO$_2$. The authors concluded that the Invos device mainly measured extracerebral tissue oxygenation. However, this conclusion must be discussed in the light of the fact that the optodes of the new Invos probes are 3.0 and 4.0 cm apart from each other. Since penetration of the cranium increases with optode distance, the new Invos probe can be assumed to accurately measure the changes of intracerebral tissue oxygenation. The use of transcranial Doppler sonography, however, as a reference method is highly questionable, because no study has validated that vMCA is an adequate parameter of regional cortical blood flow (3, 53).

Germon et al. (18) studied the effects of extracranial ischemia and intracranial hypoxia on regional cerebral oxygen saturation and demonstrated that rSO_2 is at least partially influenced by extracranial oxygen saturation. Further criticism was brought up by Brown et al. (7) who compared rSO_2 and jugular venous oxygen saturation in nine patients undergoing cardiac surgery. They found that the method of cerebral oximetry was less accurate and precise than the measurement of oxygen saturation in jugular venous blood.

In summary, although near infrared spectroscopy is capable to sensitively detect cerebral ischemia, further validation is necessary to define the precise treshold indicating cerebral ischemia by NIRS. It should be kept in mind that rSO_2 is dependent on a variety of different factors, including the distribution of blood within the vascular bed, the cerebral oxygen consumption and the oxyhemoglobin dissociation curve, respectively. For further evaluation of the significance of near infrared spectroscopy, we suggest the simultaneous measurement of rSO_2, SSEP, jugularvenous oxygen saturation and metabolites of the energy metabolism.

Invasive monitoring of cerebral perfusion with jugular bulb catheter

Measurement of jugular venous oxygen saturation is an on-line monitoring of the relationship between cerebral oxygen delivery and oxygen consumption which should facilitate the immediate detection of cerebral ischemia and the control of therapeutic interventions (35). The changes of oxygen saturation in the jugular bulb can be continuously measured with fiberoptic catheters. According to the Fick principle, measurement of arterial-jugular oxygen content difference ($AjDO_2$) allows some estimation of the relationship between cerebral metabolic rate and cerebral blood flow. If cerebral oxygen consumption, hemoglobin level, SaO_2 and the position of the hemoglobin dissociation curve remain constant, jugular venous oxygen saturation changes in proportion to cerebral blood flow (19, 35, 37).

In the absence of anemia or a sudden increase in SaO_2, a rise in SjO_2 over 75 % ($AJDO_2$ < 4 ml/100 ml blood) indicates relative (CBF < 40 ml/min/100 g) or absolute (CBF > 40 ml/min/100 g) hyperemia. This is called luxury perfusion. A decrease of SjO_2 below 50 % ($AJDO_2$ > 7.5 ml/100 ml blood) suggests relative hypoperfusion. If SjO_2 falls below 40 % and $AJDO_2$ rises above 9.0 ml/100 ml blood, global cerebral ischemia is likely (10). Severe head injury, subarachnoidal and intracerebral bleeding, cardiac surgery and cardiopulmonary resuscitation are clear indications to monitor jugular venous oxygen saturation.

Jugular bulb venous oxygen saturation monitoring seems to be an unsuitable method to detect focal cerebral ischemia. Dinkel et al. (12) found no difference in jugular venous oxygen saturation in patients with and without loss of SSEP.

Limitations of monitoring jugular venous oxygen saturation

SjO_2 reflects the relationship between cerebral blood flow and cerebral oxygen consumption. Quantification of cerebral blood flow is not possible. It is important to note that normal SjO_2 does not exclude focal cerebral ischemia. Contraindications to introduce a jugular bulb catheter are: hemorrhargic diathesis, local infection, and impaired venous blood flow (10). Inadvertent carotid puncture has occurred in 3 % (19).

References

1. Astrup J, Symon L, Branston NM, Lassen NA (1977) Cortical evoked potential and extracellular K^+ and H^+ at critical levels of brain ischemia. Stroke 8: 51–57
2. Bashein G, Nessly ML, Bledsoe SW, Townes BD, Davis KB, Coppel DB, Hornbein TF (1992) Electroencephalography during surgery with cardiopulmonary bypass and hypothermia. Anesthesiology 76: 878–891
3. Black S, Mahla ME, Cucchiara RF (1994) Neurologic monitoring. In: Miller RD (ed) Anesthesia. Fourth Edition, Churchill Livingstone Inc., New York Edinburgh Melbourne Milan Tokyo, pp 1319–1344
4. Branston NM, Symon L, Crockard HA, Pasztor E (1974) Relationship between the cortical evoked potential and local cortical blood flow following acute middle cerebral artery occlusion in the baboon. Exp Neurol 45: 195–208
5. Branston NM, Symon L, Crockard HA (1976) Recovery of the cortical evoked response following temporary middle cerebral artery occlusion in baboons: relation to local blood flow and PO_2. Stroke 7: 151–157
6. Brazy JE (1991) Near-infrared spectroscopy. Clinics in Perinatology 18: 519–534
7. Brown R, Wright G, Royston D (1993) A comparison of two systems for assessing cerebral venous oxyhaemoglobin saturation during cardiopulmonary bypass in humans. Anaesthesia 48: 697–700
8. Claus D (1994) Anatomie und Physiologie der zentralnervösen afferenten und efferenten Reizleitung. In: Rügheimer E, Dinkel M (eds) Klinische Anästhesiologie und Intensivtherapie – Neuromonitoring in Anästhesie und Intensivmedizin – vol. 46. Springer Verlag, Berlin Heidelberg New York London Paris Tokyo Hong Kong Barcelona Budapest, pp 3–16
9. Craft RM, Losasso TJ, Perkins WJ, Weglinski MR, Sharbrough FW (1994) EEG monitoring for cerebral ischemia during carotid endarterectomy (CEA): How much is enough? Anesthesiology 81: A214
10. Dearden NM (1994) Jugular bulb venous oxygen saturation and transcranial doppler ultrasonography in neurosurgical patients. In: Schulte am Esch, Kochs E (eds) Central nervous system monitoring in anesthesia and intensive care. Springer Verlag, Berlin Heidelberg New York London Paris Tokyo Hong Kong Barcelona Budapest, pp 292–313
11. Dinkel M (1994) Neurophysiologisches Monitoring in der perioperativen Phase: Grundlagen und Problematik. In: Rügheimer E, Dinkel M (eds) Klinische Anästhesiologie und Intensivtherapie – Neuromonitoring in Anästhesie und Intensivmedizin – vol. 46. Springer Verlag, Berlin Heidelberg New York London Paris Tokyo Hong Kong Barcelona Budapest, pp 111–123
12. Dinkel M, Lörler H, Langer H, Schweiger H, Rügheimer E (1994) Evoked potential monitoring for vascular surgery. In: Schulte am Esch, Kochs E (eds) Central nervous system monitoring in anesthesia and intensive care. Springer Verlag, Berlin Heidelberg New York London Paris Tokyo Hong Kong Barcelona Budapest, pp 230–247
13. Drummond JC, Todd MM, Sang H (1985) The effect of high dose sodium thiopental on brain stem auditory and median nerve somatosensory evoked responses in humans. Anesthesiology 63: 249–254
14. Drummond JC, Shapiro HM (1994) Cerebral physiology. In: Miller RD (ed) Anesthesia. Fourth Edition, Churchill Livingstone Inc., New York Edinburgh Melbourne Milan Tokyo, pp 689–729
15. Edmonds HL, Griffiths LK, van der Laken J, Slater AD, Shields CB (1992) Quantitative electroencephalographic monitoring during myocardial revascularization predicts postoperative disorientation and improves outcome. J Thorac Cardiovasc Surg 103: 555–563
16. Edwards AD, Richardson C, Zee van der P, Elwell C, Wyatt JS, Cope M, Delpy DT, Reynolds EOR (1993) Measurement of hemoglobin flow and blood flow by near-infrared spectroscopy. J Appl Physiol 75: 1884–1889

17. Engelhardt W (1994) Neurophysiologisches Monitoring bei kardiochirurgischen Eingriffen. In: Rügheimer E, Dinkel M (eds) Klinische Anästhesiologie und Intensivtherapie – Neuromonitoring in Anästhesie und Intensivmedizin – vol. 46. Springer Verlag, Berlin Heidelberg New York London Paris Tokyo Hong Kong Barcelona Budapest, pp 201–207
18. Germon TJ, Kane NM, Manara AR, Nelson RJ (1994) Near-infrared spectroscopy in adults: effects of extracranial ischemia and intracranial hypoxia on estimation of cerebral oxygenation. Br J Anaesth 73: 503–506
19. Goetting MG, Preston G (1990) Jugular bulb catherization: Experience with 123 patients. Crit Care Med 18: 1220
20. Greenfield JC Jr, Rembert JC, Tindall GT (1984) Transient changes in cerebral vascular resistance during the Valsalva maneuver in man. Stroke 15: 76–79
21. Grundy BL, Heros RC, Tung AS, Doyle E (1981) Intraoperative hypoxia detected by evoked potential monitoring. Anesth Analg 60: 437–439
22. Harris DNF, Bailey SM (1993) Near infrared spectroscopy in adults. Does the Invos 3100 really measure intracerebral oxygenation? Anaesthesia 48: 694–696
23. Jobsis FF (1977) Noninvasive, infrared monitoring of cerebral and myocardial oxygen sufficiency and circulatory parameters. Science 198: 1264–1267
24. Johansson BB, Auer LM (1983) Neurogenic modification of the vulnerability of the blood-brain-barrier during hypertension in conscious rats. Acta Physiol Scand 117: 507–511
25. Kety S, Schmidt CF (1945) The determination of cerebral blood flow in man by the use of nitrous oxide in low concentrations. Am J Physiol 143: 53–66
26. Kochs E, Bischoff P (1994) Anesthesia and somatosensory evoked responses. In: Schulte am Esch, Kochs E (eds) Central nervous system monitoring in anesthesia and intensive care. Springer Verlag, Berlin Heidelberg New York London Paris Tokyo Hong Kong Barcelona Budapest, pp 146–175
27. Koht A, Schütz W, Schmidt G, Schramm J, Watanabe E (1988) Effects of etomidat, midazolam, and thiopental on median nerve somatosensory evoked potentials and the additive effects of fentanyl and nitrous oxide. Anesth Analg 67: 435–441
28. Kurth CD, Steven JM, Nicolson SC, Chance B, Delivoria-Papadopoulos M (1992) Kinetics of cerebral deoxygenation during deep hypothermic circulatory arrest in neonates. Anesthesiology 77: 656–661
29. Lam AM, Manninen PH, Ferguson GG, Nantau W (1991) Monitoring electrophysiologic function during carotid endarterectomy: A comparison of somatosensory evoked potentials and conventional electroencephalogram. Anesthesiology 75: 15–21
30. Langer H, Lörler H, Singer W, Dinkel M (1994) Objektivierung kritischer regionaler Hirnischämien durch computergestützte topographische Elektroenzephalometrie. Anaesthesist (Suppl 1) 43: 165 FV 18.8
31. Levy WJ (1987) Effect of epoch length on power spectrum analysis of the EEG. Anesthesiology 66: 489–495
32. Lou HC, Edvinsson L, MacKenzie ET (1987) The concept of coupling blood flow to brain function: revision required? Ann Neurol 22: 289–297
33. Matsumoto H, Oda T, Hossain MA, Yoshimura N (1994) Monitoring of cytochrom aa3 reduction by near infrared spectrophotometry reflects brain energy depletion during hypoxia. Anesthesiology 81: A528
34. McCormick PW, Stewart M, Goetting MG, Dujovny M, Lewis G, Ausman JI (1991) Noninvasive cerebral optical spectroscopy for monitoring cerebral oxygen delivery and hemodynamics. Crit Care Med 19: 89–97
35. Metz Ch, Bein TH, Reng M, Taeger K (1993) Die zerebrovenöse Oxymetrie bei Patienten mit Schädel-Hirn-Verletzungen. Anästh Intensivmed 34: 345–355
36. Mintun MA, Raichle ME, Martin WR, Herscovitch P (1984) Brain oxygen utilization measured with O-15 radiotracers and positron emission tomography. J Nucl Med 25: 177–187
37. Murr R (1994) Zerebrales Monitoring bei Schädel-Hirn-Trauma. Anästh Intensivmed 35: 229–309
38. Nollert G, Tassani-Prell P, Möhnle P, Uttner I, Schmoeckel M, Reichart B (1994) Monitoring of brain activity and oxygenation during cardiac operations. J Cardiothoracic Vascular Anesthesia 8 (Suppl) 3: 67
39. Pathak KS, Amaddio MD, Scoles PV, Shaffer JW, Mackay W (1989) Effects of halothane, enflurane, and isoflurane in nitrous oxide on multilevel somatosensory evoked potentials. Anesthesiology 70: 207–212
40. Peterson DO, Drummond JC, Todd MM (1986) Effects of halothane, isoflurane, and nitrous oxide on somatosensory evoked potentials in humans. Anesthesiology 65: 35–40
41. Russ W, Kling D, Loesevitz A, Hempelman G (1984) Effect of hypothermia on visual evoked potentials (VEP) in humans. Anesthesiology 61: 207–210
42. Samra SK, Vanderzant CW, Domer PA, Sackellares C (1987) Differential effects of isoflurane on human median nerve somatosensory evoked potentials. Anesthesiology 66: 29–35
43. Schregel W (1994) Die Bedeutung der transkraniellen Dopplersonographie als nichtinvasives Untersuchungsverfahren in Anästhesie und Intensivmedizin. In: Rügheimer E, Dinkel M (eds) Klinische Anästhesiologie und Intensivtherapie – Neuromonitoring in Anästhesie und Intensivmedizin – vol. 46. Springer Verlag, Berlin Heidelberg New York London Paris Tokyo Hong Kong Barcelona Budapest, pp 104–110

44. Schüttler J (1994) EEG-Monitoring zur Quantifizierung der „Narkosetiefe": Möglichkeiten und Grenzen. In: Rügheimer E, Dinkel M (eds) Klinische Anästhesiologie und Intensivtherapie – Neuromonitoring in Anästhesie und Intensivmedizin – vol. 46. Springer Verlag, Berlin Heidelberg New York London Paris Tokyo Hong Kong Barcelona Budapest, pp 306–318

45. Schwender D, Golling W, Klasing S, Faber-Züllig E, Pöppel E, Peter K (1994) Effects of surgical stimulation on midlatency auditory evoked potentials during general anaesthesia with propofol/fentanyl, isoflurane/fentanyl and flunitrazepam/fentanyl. Anaesthesia 49: 572–578

46. Smith JJ, Hudetz AG, Lee JG, Bosnjak ZJ, Kampine JP (1994) Cerebrocortical laser Doppler flow response to CO_2: preserved after nitric oxide synthase inhibition in the rat? Anesthesiology 81: A690

47. Sokoloff L (1981) Schmitt Lecture in Neuroscience 1980. The relationship between function and energy metabolism: its use in the localization of functional activity in the nervous system. Neurosci-Res-Program-Bull 19: 159–207

48. Sylvia AL, Piantadosi CA, Jobsis-Vander-Vliet FF (1985) Energy metabolism and in vivo cytochrom c oxidase redox relationships in hypoxic rat brain. Neurol Res 7: 81–88

49. Symon L (1985) Flow thresholds in brain ischemia and the effects of drugs. Br J Anaesth 57: 34–43

50. Tamura M, Hazeki O, Nioka S, Chance B, Smith DS (1988) The simultaneous measurements of tissue oxygen concentration and energy state by near infrared and nuclear magnetic resonance spectroscopy. Adv-Exp-Med-Biol 222: 359–363

51. Thornton C, Creagh-Barry P, Newton DEF (1994) Peri-operative anesthesiological monitoring of auditory-evoked potentials. In: Schulte am Esch, Kochs E (eds) Central nervous system monitoring in anesthesia and intensive care. Springer Verlag, Berlin Heidelberg New York London Paris Tokyo Hong Kong Barcelona Budapest, pp 176–186

52. Werner C, Kochs E (1994) Monitoring of the central nervous system. Current Opinion in Anaesthesiology 7: 401–408

53. Williams IM, Picton AJ, Hardy SC, Mortimer AJ, McCollum (1994) Cerebral hypoxia detected by near infrared spectroscopy. Anaesthesia 49: 762–766

54. Wyatt JS, Cope M, Delpy DT, Richardson CE, Edwards AD, Wray S, Reynolds EOR (1990) Quantitation of cerebral blood volume in human infants by near-infrared spectroscopy. J Appl Physiol 68: 1086–1091

Author's address:
Prof. Dr. H. J. Bardenheuer
Department of Anesthesiology
University of Heidelberg
Im Neuenheimer Feld 110
69120 Heidelberg, Germany

Electroencephalography: recording technique, pathophysiological comments, intraoperative monitoring

U. Schauseil-Zipf

University Hospital for Sick Children, Cologne

Introduction

Today advanced neuroimaging techniques, transcranial Doppler ultrasound, and evoked potentials provide essential information on brain morphology and pathophysiology.

These investigations, however, can not provide nor replace the prompt and functional message from the cerebral cortex given by electroencephalography. Therefore, the EEG remains to be a valuable diagnostic tool in many medical fields. In vascular surgery, particularly in carotid surgery, electroencephalography is used to assess the function of the cerebral cortex before, during, and after operation.

Recording technique

A standard EEG investigation is carried out over a period of 20–30 minutes in either wakefulness or sleep using standard provocation methods such as hyperventilation and photic stimulation. During polysomnography the EEG is simultaneously recorded with physiological parameters such as heart rate, respiration, or oxygen saturation. Patients with sleep disorders and babies with apnoeic spells can be identified by this method.

A long-term EEG recording can be performed either ambulatory or on the patient's bed side. On an ambulatory basis it is a convenient secondary investigation for patients with epilepsy. Telemetry or magnetic tapes are used to record the analogue EEG for several hours up to several days (2). Bed side EEG monitoring is applied in patients with more severe seizure disorders as well as during intensive care treatment. The bed side EEG can be evaluated either as an analogue "on line" record or after computerized processing by frequency analysis. From the technical point of view the intraoperative EEG monitoring during neurosurgery, cardiac surgery, and vascular surgery does not differ from the intensive care EEG monitoring. EEG and evoked potentials are often simultaneously recorded in the operating theater and evaluated by a neurophysiologist (4, 6).

Pathophysiological comments

Regarding the diagnostic value of electroencephalography, it is important to know that EEG abnormalities reflect general pathophysiological processes, for example, epileptogenesis or encephalopathy. However, EEG abnormalities in most instances show little or no specificity for a particular disease. Consequently the abnormal EEG has to be interpreted together with the actual clinical context to get satisfactory diagnostic information.

Maturation of the cerebral cortex from birth to adulthood changes the traces of the EEG significantly. In seizure disorders paroxysmal activity can be seen in various patterns, thus, confirming the diagnosis of epilepsy. Functional and structural focal brain lesions can be demonstrated by electroencephalography even in cases where MRT and CT scans fail to show focal abnormalities. Diffuse encephalopathy, for example, hypoxic ischemic encephalopathy during or after vascular surgery, alters the EEG dramatically and the clinical course of the encephalopathic process can be monitored by follow up EEG investigations. Diagnostic information of the EEG can be obtained in patients with organic brain syndromes and dementias, in comatose patients, and for the evaluation of brain death. Furthermore, the EEG is a useful investigation for the diagnostic approach to sleep disorders (1).

Drug effects can alter the EEG remarkably, for example, in patients with diazepam medication. Depending on the duration of diazepam intake the EEG shows an excess of fast activity for hours, days or weeks after the end of drug administration. Similarly, general anesthesia has significant effects on the electroencephalogramm: during deepening general anesthesia the EEG shows a sequence of alterations that parallel the increasing depression of cerebral oxygen metabolism. The overall electric output declines gradually after an initial transient increase. There is, however, no simple linear relationship between anesthetic depth and level of cerebral activity (4). Therefore, no consensus has emerged as to the reliability of perioperative EEG measures in determining the depth of anesthesia.

Intraoperative EEG monitoring

As mentioned before, important clinical information can be obtained from EEG monitoring in the operating theater and in the intensive care unit, where patients may experience a decline in cerebral blood flow related to increased intracranial pressure or other ischemic events. It is the goal of continous EEG monitoring to recognize a decline in the patient's condition before physical signs and symptoms are present and, in addition, to provide reliable prognostic information. Consequently, EEG monitoring can help to avoid either untertreatment and overtreatment in the intensive care unit (5, 6).

Intraoperative EEG monitoring has become a standard technique in cardiac surgery, neurosurgery, and vascular surgery. Analogue and computerized EEG recordings during carotid surgery show alterations of cortical funtion due to cerebral ischemia soon after carotid clamping. EEG abnormalities occur as soon as carotid clamping reduces the cerebral blood flow to 18–24 ml/100 g/min or less. Amplitude changes of the EEG and the evoked potentials appear to be more important than frequency shifts during clamping. Both, EEG and EP abnormalities are reversed by shunting (4, 7).

A major tool in EEG monitoring is the compressed spectral array (CSA). By "piling up" spectra on a vertical line, one can visualize frequency spectral characteristics of an EEG channel over long periods of time (6). It is thus possible to follow gradual changes in spectral components by comparing early and later parts of the display. However, no information can be obtained about the amplitude of the EEG activity, which is very sensitive to alterations of cerebral blood flow. There are different opinions concerning the sensitivity of CSA. Recent studies by Kearse et al. (3) indicate that CSA does not reliably detect mild analogue EEG pattern changes of cerebral ischemia and is, therefore, not a reliable substitute for analogue EEG monitoring during carotid endarterectomy. Both analogue and digitized EEG recording techniques should be available in the operating room during cardiac and vascular surgery as well as during neurosurgery procedures.

Conclusion

High technological standards and an individual problem solving approach are necessary for an effective and reliable EEG service. Intraoperative EEG monitoring during vascular surgery allows immediate recognition of impaired cerebral function at a stage before irreversible damage occurs. Monitoring the functional state of the brain by EEG and evoked potentials has a significant role in the prevention of postoperative neurological complications and helps to improve the quality of patient care.

References

1. Daly DD, Pedley TA (eds) (1990) Current Practise of Clinical Electroencephalography. Second Edition, Raven Press, New York
2. Ebersole JS (1989) Ambulatory EEG Monitoring, Raven Press, New York
3. Kearse LA Jr, Brown EN, McPeck K (1992) Somatosensory evoked potentials sensitivity relative to electroencephalography for cerebral ischemia during carotid endarterectomy. Stroke 23: 498–505
4. Loftus CM, Traynelis VC (1994) Intraoperative Monitoring Techniques in Neurosurgery, Mc Graw-Hill, Inc New York, St Louis, San Francisco, Auckland, Bogota, Caracas, Lisbon, London, Madrid, Mexico City, Milan, Montreal, New Dehli, Paris, San Juan, Singapore, Sydney, Tokyo, Toronto
5. Lopes Da Silva FH, Storm van Leeuwen W, Remond A (1986) Clinical Applications of Computer Analysis of EEG and other Neurophysiological Signals, Handbook of Electroencephalography and Clinical Neurophysiology. Vol 2 Elsevier, Amsterdam, New York, Oxford
6. Prior PF, Douglas EM (1986) Monitoring Cerebral Function. Long-Term Monitoring of EEG and Evoked Potentials. Elsevier, Amsterdam, New York, Oxford
7. Schramm J, Moller AR (eds) (1991) Intraoperative Neurophysiologic Monitoring in Neurosurgery. Springer Verlag, Berlin, Heidelberg, New York, London, Paris, Tokyo, Hong Kong, Barcelona, Budapest

Author's address:
Priv.-Doz. Dr. U. Schauseil-Zipf
University Hospital for Sick Children Cologne
Joseph-Stelzmann-Str. 9
50924 Köln, Germany

Monitoring of somatosensory evoked potentials in carotid artery surgery

W. F. Haupt[1], S. Horsch[2]

[1] Department of Neurology, University of Cologne, Cologne, Germany
[2] Department of Surgery, Krankenhaus Porz, Cologne, Germany

Introduction

The surgical treatment of high-grade extracranial stenosis of the carotid artery has been shown to reduce the incidence of cerebral vascular disease (4, 13). This elective and prophylactic surgical treatment must meet high quality standards with respect to preoperative diagnostics and operative management to be of benefit to the patient. Operations on arteries supplying the brain must be considered high-risk procedures and should therefore be performed with the highest possible level of security. Intraoperative monitoring of brain function is desirable since neurological complications cannot be detected intraoperatively by clinical examination. These monitoring methods should be reasonably simple to perform, sensitive, reliable, and cost effective. The method of median-nerve evoked somatosensory evoked potentials (SEP) fulfills these requirements.

Method

Somatosensory evoked potentials are generated by the afferent somatosensory nerve fibers leading from the periphery of extremities to the cortical somatosensory projection areas of the brain cortex which are located in the postcentral gyrus of the parietal lobe.

Peripheral nerves are stimulated by electrical impulses, and the evoked responses are registered by surface electrodes. Since the amplitude of the responses is in the order of about 2–10 µV, special electronic averaging procedures are necessary to obtain a favorable signal-noise ratio. Usually, one has to average between 200 and 1000 individual stimulus responses to obtain a reliable evoked response.

The evoked potentials can be registered at various sites along the somatosensory pathways. In the case of median-nerve evoked SEPs, typical registration sites are in the supraclavicular fossa, over the cervical spine at C7 and C2, and over the cortical somatosensory representation area of the parietal cortex (Fig. 1). The cortical registration is performed at the positions C4' for the right hemisphere and C3' for the left hemisphere with a reference electrode at Fz (Fig. 2). Tibial nerve SEP can be registered in the popliteal fossa, over the lumbar spine at L5, the cervical spine at C7, and the cerebral cortex.

For purposes of intraoperative monitoring in carotid artery surgery, median-nerve evoked potentials are especially well suited since the evoked response is generated by the somatosensory cortex in the parietal lobe, an area which is supplied by the middle cerebral artery. This main brain artery is supplied exclusively by the internal carotid artery. Therefore, critical perfusion deficits in the common or internal carotid arteries have a direct effect on the perfusion of the middle cerebral artery, leading to immediate functional disturbances of the parietal lobe and the somatosensory projection area in the postcentral gyrus (Fig. 2). Median-nerve SEP therefore reflect the functional status of the carotid artery. Animal experiments and clinical data have shown that a critical lowering of perfusion in the somatosensory projection area leads to immediate changes of SEP (2). For this reason, median-nerve evoked potentials render a reliable tool to monitor the function of cerebral perfusion. In carotid artery surgery, intact peripheral and spinal somatosensory pathways can be assumed and proven by preoperative median-nerve evoked SEP registrations. For this reason, it is sufficient to register only cortical SEP responses during operations. Although SEP registrations only reflect the functional status of the postcentral somatosensory area, this area is representative of the whole supply area of the middle cerebral artery and therefore sufficient for monitoring purposes. For intraoperative monitoring purposes, it is sufficient to determine the latency of the main cortical evoked response, the N 20 wave. A prolongation of the latency beyond the 2.5 standard deviation of predeter-

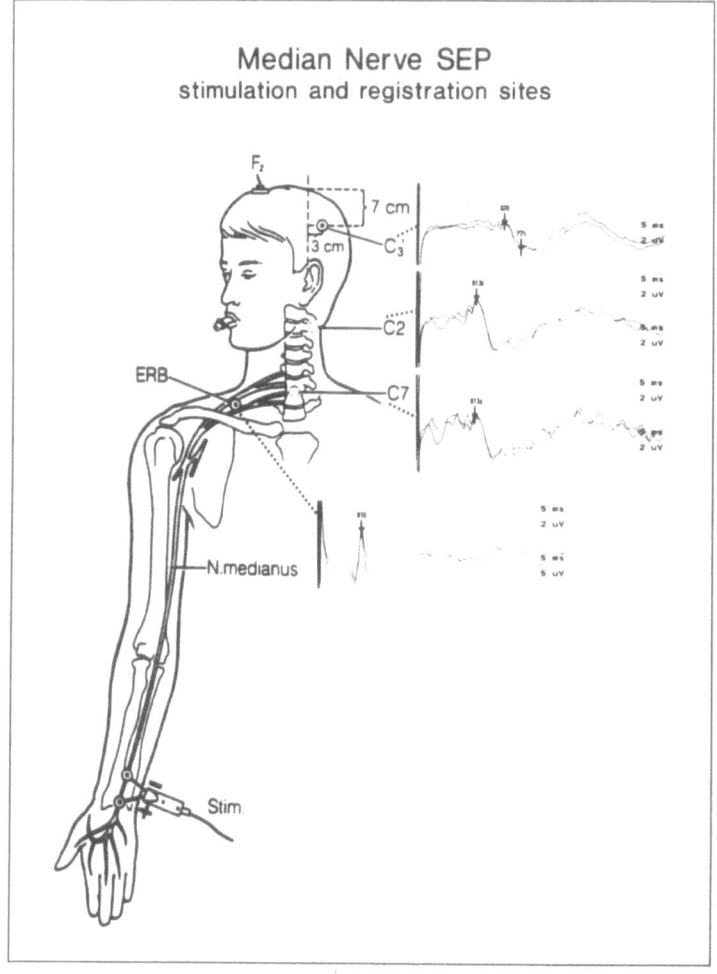

Fig. 1.

mined standard values is considered significant. Reductions of the N20/P25 amplitude of more than 50 % of the baseline preoperative value are also considered significant.

Almost all inhalation and intravenous anesthetic agents such as halothane, enflurane, N_2O, fentanyl, propofol and others lead to amplitude changes of SEP. However, these effects are minor and much less pronounced than the effect on EEG activity. Usual concentrations of these agents during anesthesia do not interfere with SEP monitoring. We prefer the use of fentanyl and propofol or droperidol and isoflurane which has the least effect on the amplitude of SEP.

The electrophysiological testing apparatus is small enough to not interfere with the operation.

Results

In our series of 994 operations, we attempted SEP monitoring in all cases. No clearly resolved SEP could be obtained in 9.9 % of the cases. In 78.7 % of the procedures, we observed

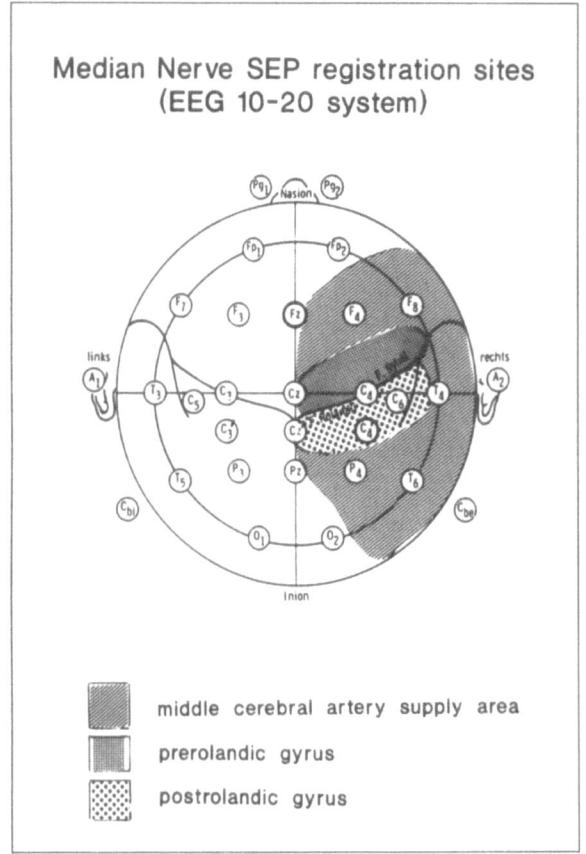

Fig. 2.

no changes of the SEP, in 10.5 % of the cases, we encountered reversible changes of the SEP amplitude. In 0.7 % of the operations, we found irreversible loss of SEP over the corresponding hemisphere which was associated with new irreversible neurological deficit in all cases. In only one case, we found a new neurological deficit without intraoperative changes of the SEP. Hence, the sensitivity of SEP monitoring for the prediction of complications was 87 % for the total number of complications or 99.9 % with respect to the total number of operations. No mortalities occurred during or after the operations. Figure 3 demonstrates the registration of SEP during an operation without any changes and without postoperative complications. Figure 4 shows reversible SEP amplitude changes during cross-clamping of the carotid artery in the presence of significant stenosis of the contra-lateral carotid artery indicating poor collateralization of the cerebral blood supply. Figure 5 shows acute intraoperative SEP loss indicating embolic infarction of the dependent hemisphere (1, 5, 7, 8, 11).

Although only limited therapeutic options are available during operation in the light of acute SEP loss indicating brain infarction, the surgeon and anesthesiologist should be informed of the event and should attempt to complete the procedure as soon as possible

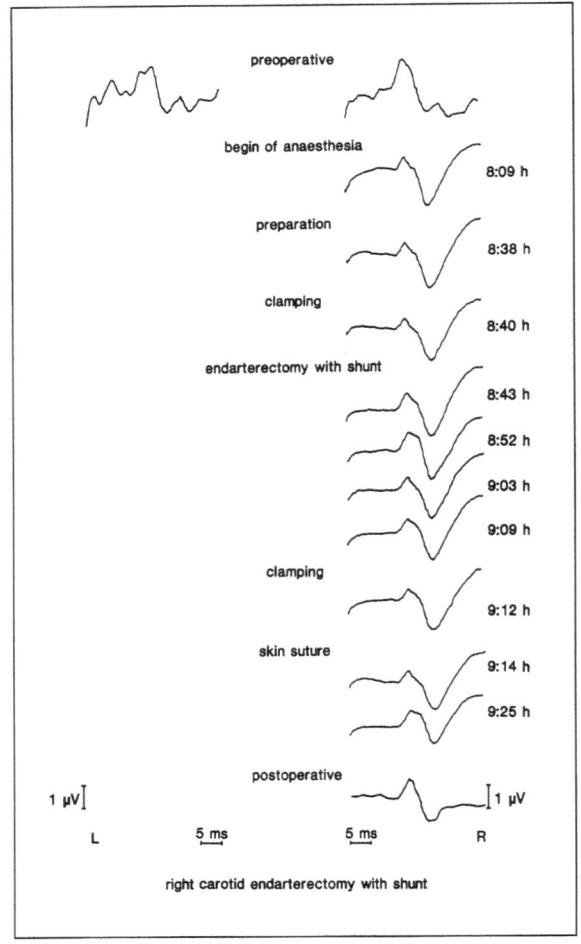

Fig. 3.

and optimize the cardiovascular situation. The patient should be admitted to an ICU immediately after the operation and treated for brain infarction.

In a single case outside of this series, we encountered a patient who developed marked right-sided hemiparesis and aphasia following left carotid endarterectomy. The SEP recordings showed no pre-, intra-, or postoperative changes. Serial postoperative CT scans of the brain demonstrated a watershed-type infarction in the border area between the supply regions of the middle and anterior cerebral arteries which could be attributed to a hemodynamic infarction due to a significant blood pressure drop in the induction phase of anesthesia. This rare situation of infarction in the fronto-parietal brain region could not be detected by single-channel EP recordings over the parietal lobe. Perhaps multiple-channel recordings from the postrolandic and prerolandic regions could have detected this complication which would involve a higher technical expenditure (5, 9, 10, 15).

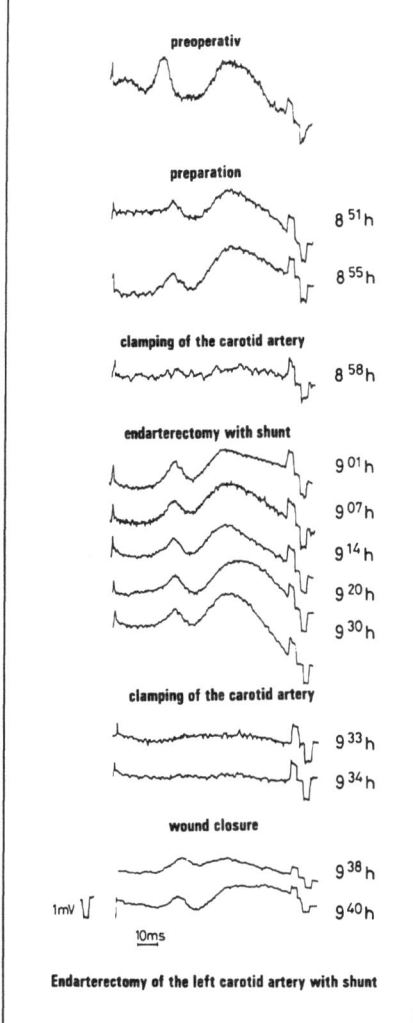

Fig. 4.

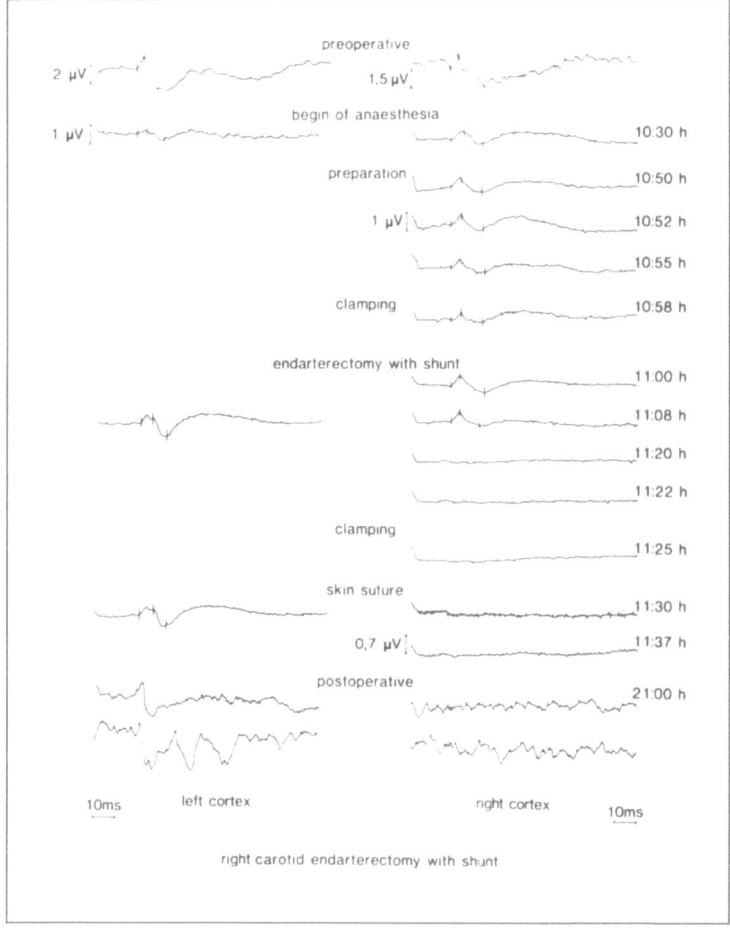

Fig. 5.

Discussion

According to the results of the literature (1, 5, 11) and our own results (7, 8) in a large series of patients, monitoring of carotid endarterectomies with SEP has proven to be a safe and reliable method. Although only a small region of the brain is monitored for functional disturbance, the data are sufficient to reliably assess critical changes of perfusion in the relevant brain area. The use of only one recording channel makes the procedure simple to handle. The monitored data is reduced to one latency and amplitude measurement. The method can be performed by a technician after a short training period. The necessary electrophysiological equipment is no more expensive than conventional EEG equipment and is therefore cost-effective. The method is much less elaborate than conventional EEG monitoring which requires between 10 and 21 recording electrodes. Moreover, the interpretation of EEG recordings is much more complex and requires a significantly higher degree of training especially with respect to the detection of artifacts (3, 6, 12, 16, 17).

Various computerized EEG monitoring systems using a digitalized EEG spectral analysis have been developed which are rather prone to problems concerning artifacts and seem to have a higher rate of false-positive findings (14).

References

1. Amantini A, Bartelli M, de Scisciolo G, Lombardi M, Rossi R, Pratesi C, Pinto F (1992) Monitoring of somatosensory evoked potentials during carotid endarterectomy. J Neurol 239: 241–247
2. Branston NM, Symon L, Crockard HA, Prasztor E (1974) Relationship between the cortical evoked potential and local cortical blood flow following acute middle cerebral artery occlusion in the baboon. Exp Neurol 45: 195–208
3. Chiappa KH, Burke SR, Young RR (1979) Results of electroencephalographic monitoring during 367 carotid endarterectomies. Stroke 10: 381–388
4. European Carotid Surgery Triallists' Collaborative Group (1991) MRC european carotid surgery trial: interim results for symptomatic patients with severe (70–99 %) or with mild (0–29 %) carotid stenosis. Lancet 337: 1235–1243
5. Gigli GL, Caramia M, Marciani MG, Zarola F, Lavaroni F, Rossini PM (1987) Monitoring of subcortical and cortical somatosensory evoked potentials during carotid endarterectomy: comparison with stump pressure levels. Electroenceph Clin Neurophysiol 68: 424–432
6. Harris EJ, Brown WH, Pavy RN, Anderson WW, Stone DW (1967) Continuous electroencephalographic monitoring during carotid artery endarterectomy. Surgery 62: 441–447
7. Haupt WF, de Vleeschauwer P, Horsch S (1985) Veränderungen somatosensibel evozierter Potentiale während Karotis-Desobliteration. Diagnostische Bedeutung und mögliche Konsequenzen für die Therapie. Z EEG-EMG 16: 201–205
8. Haupt WF, Horsch S (1992) Evoked potential monitoring in carotid surgery: a review of 994 cases. Neurology (Minneap) 42: 835–838
9. Haupt WF, Erasmi-Körber H, Lanfermann H (1994) Intraoperative recording of parietal SEP can miss hemodynamic infarction during carotid endarterectomy: a case study. Electroenceph Clin Neurophysiol 92: 86–88
10. Krul JMJ, van Gijn J, Ackerstaff RGA, Eikelboom BC, Theorides T, Vermeulen FEE (1989) Site and pathogenesis of infarcts associated with carotid endarterectomy. Stroke 20: 324–328
11. Markand ON, Dilley RS, Moorthy SS, Warren C (1984) Monitoring of somatosensory evoked responses during carotid endarterectomy. Arch Neurol 41: 375–378
12. Mola M, Collice M, Levati A (1986) Continuous intraoperative electroencephalographic monitoring in carotid endarterectomy. Eur Neurol 25: 53–60
13. North American Symptomatic Carotid Endarterectomy Trial Collaborators (1991) Beneficial effect of carotid endarterectomy in symptomatic patients with high-grade carotid stenosis. New Engl J Med 325: 445–453
14. Rampil IJ, Holzer JA, Quest DO, Rosenbaum SH, Correll JW (1983) Prognostic value of computerized EEG analysis during carotid endarterectomy. Anesth Analg 62: 186–192
15. Ringelstein EB, Zeumer H, Schneider R (1985) Der Beitrag der zerebralen Computertomographie zur Differentialtypologie und Differentialtherapie des ischämischen Großhirninfarktes. Fortschr Neurol Psychiat 53: 315–336
16. Sundt TM, Sharbrough FW, Piepgras DG, Kearns TP, Messick JM, O'Fallon WM (1981) Correlation of cerebral blood flow and electroencephalographic changes during carotid endarterectomy. Mayo Clin Proc 56: 533–543
17. Trojaborg W, Boysen G (1973) Relation between EEG, regional cerebral blood flow and internal carotid artery pressure during carotid endarterectomy. Electroenceph Clin Neurophysiol 34: 61–69

Author's address:
Prof. Dr. W. F. Haupt, MD
Clinic of Neurology and Psychiatry
of the University of Cologne
Josef-Stelzmann-Str. 9
50924 Köln, Germany

Internal carotid artery back pressure to determine shunt requirement

W. S. Moore

Section of Vascular Surgery, UCLA Center for the Health Sciences, Los Angeles, CA, USA

Introduction

During the early experience with carotid endarterectomy, performed under local anesthesia, it was noted that there was a small percentage of patients who would develop a prompt neurologic deficit when the carotid artery was clamped in preparation for arteriotomy and endarterectomy. This occurred in approximately 10 % of patients, and the deficit could be promptly reversed with the placement of an internal shunt. It was generally assumed that this small but identifiable group of patients had inadequate collateral circulation in the distribution of the clamped artery. Therefore, collaterals were insufficient to provide for blood flow during the carotid endarterectomy. It was further assumed that to continue the operation without the use of an internal shunt would inevitably result in ischemic brain damage and probable cerebral infarction in the affected hemisphere. While it is easy to identify the patient who needs a shunt under local anesthesia, this was not so under general anesthesia. Since there was an increasing trend to perform this operation under general anesthesia, the surgeons at that time were left with little choice but to do all carotid endarterectomies with an internal shunt. A shunt was regarded as being an additional step in the operation. At best it was a cumbersome inconvenience. At worst it was a source of additional risk from arterial injury or from cerebral embolization with either air bubbles or atheromatous debris. Attempts were made to identify the small but finite percentage of patients who would require a shunt. Selective shunting could be used in those patients with inadequate collateral blood flow in order to protect them from ischemic brain damage during clamping. Shunts and shunt-related complications could be avoided in the vast majority of patients with adequate collateral blood flow. Several methods were tried and found to be unsuccessful in their ability to accurately predict the patient who would require internal shunting. The use of carotid artery back pressure was the first successful hemodynamic test to be employed and continues to be used in some centers. It has been largely replaced, in most centers, by continuous EEG monitoring, somatosensory evoked potential measurement, or monitoring with transcranial Doppler.

Development of the back pressure method

During the course of carotid endarterectomy, under local (cervical block) anesthesia, it was a frequently noted observation that those patients who were tolerant of temporary carotid cross-clamping exhibited brisk back bleeding from the internal carotid artery when the clamp was released. Conversely, those patients in whom carotid clamping resulted in loss of consciousness or the onset of neurologic dysfunction were found to have rather poor back bleeding when the clamp was removed from the internal carotid artery. In 1966, we decided to develop a method for identifying patients with inadequate collateral cerebral blood flow that did not depend upon the awake or conscious response of the patient undergoing carotid endarterectomy. Our objective was to identify a reliable method such that carotid endarterectomy could be performed under general anesthesia with the selective rather than the routine use of internal shunting.

The correlation between slow back bleeding from the internal carotid artery and intolerance to temporary clamping had already been appreciated and served as a basis for our early clinical experiments. Initially, we thought that we could quantitate the rate of black flow in the internal carotid artery in order to establish a threshold value, below which an internal shunt would be required and above which the operation could be performed without the aid of a shunt. Thus proved to be a rather cumbersome and time-consuming method. As an alternative, it seemed reasonable to assume that the measurement of static back pressure in the internal carotid artery should correlate with potential back flow and be an indicator of the adequacy of collateral cerebral blood flow. We decided to test this hypothesis by performing the next 48 carotid endarterectomies under local anesthesia and correlating the neurologic response to clamping with the measurement of internal carotid artery back pressure. During five operations, a temporary neurologic deficit occurred with clamping, and all of them were reversed with placement of an internal shunt. All five patients had internal carotid artery back pressure of < 25 mm Hg. Specifically, these measured 12, 14, 19, 20, and 22 mm Hg. Forty-three carotid endarterectomies were performed, during which temporary carotid clamping was well tolerated. The internal carotid artery back pressures in these patients ranged from 25 – 88 mm Hg. This seemed to be a good correlation and suggested that our hypothesis was correct. Furthermore, we established that a back pressure of 25 mm Hg was an absolute minimum. A lower pressure was an indication for shunting (11).

Validation of the back pressure method

The data from our initial clinical experiment appeared to be sufficiently compelling so that we were then prepared to proceed with the next step of validation. This involved performing the next series of carotid endarterectomies under general anesthesia, during which time a decision of whether or not to use a shunt was based upon internal carotid artery back pressure measurement. We performed 107 carotid endarterectomies in 78 patients and made the decision to shunt based upon a measured internal carotid artery back pressure of 25 mm or less. All patients with back pressures in excess of 25 mm Hg had carotid endarterectomy performed without a shunt. We then carried out an analysis of the incidence of neurologic complications as a function of indication for operation. We found that the use of internal carotid artery back pressure as a means of decision for using an internal shunt appeared to be quite accurate for those patients in whom carotid endarterectomy was being performed for either asymptomatic carotid stenosis or transient cerebral ischemia. However, the technique seemed to be less accurate for patients who had a prior stroke in the distribution of the operated artery as an indication for operation. Four of 24 patients who had experienced prior stroke as an indication for operation, with back pressures > 25 mm Hg, and in whom a shunt was not used experienced a temporary worsening of their preoperative neurologic deficit in contrast to a similar group of patients with prior stroke who had a shunt placed because of low back pressure. Those patients awoke with no worsening of the pre-existing deficit in spite of their increased risk related to poor collateral circulation. We proposed that the difference among patients who had a prior stroke in whom back pressure measurement was not a reliable measure for the adequacy of collateral cerebral blood flow and patients in whom operation was being performed for asymptomatic or transient symptoms with a very good correlation was probably related to areas of partially perfused brain surrounding the cerebral infarct, or the so-called ischemic penumbra (12). It was our recommendation, therefore, that all patients with prior stroke have routine shunting since it was difficult to know what cerebral perfusion pressure or back pressure would be required to adequately maintain nutritional blood flow to the ischemic penumbra.

Following our original publications, there have been many reports in the literature offering to either validate or refute our observations (5–9, 14). Those authors who disputed the validity of the back pressure method for determining shunt requirement would offer as their evidence an incidence of postoperative stroke in spite of a satisfactory back pressure measure. The problem with this line of reasoning is that it requires an assumption that all postoperative neurologic deficits are related to carotid clamping and inadequate cerebral blood flow. It has now been well documented that the most frequent cause of a perioperative stroke is technical and is related to thromboembolism originating from the endarterectomy site (13). Therefore, to blame a postoperative neurologic deficit upon ischemic damage caused by temporary occlusion is invalid.

Current utilization of back pressure monitoring

We continued to utilize back pressure monitoring as a means of determining shunt requirement in all patient except those who had a prior stroke as an indication for operation. With the introduction of continuous EEG monitoring, a series of reports appeared suggesting that there was poor correlation between internal carotid artery back pressure and the presence or absence of EEG change with carotid clamping (4, 9, 10). Most reports assumed, in the design of their experiment, that the presence or absence of EEG change was an absolute gold standard. Therefore, the failure of correlation between back pressure and EEG would be an indictment of the validity of back pressure measurement. We decided to carry out a series of comparisons in which we looked at the opposite hypothesis. That is, we assumed that back pressure measure would be a gold standard and determined whether or not EEG change would correlate with a poor or adequate back pressure in order to ascertain whether EEG was a valid method of measure. We carried out a series of observations in a group of patients undergoing carotid endarterectomy who had continuous EEG monitoring and in whom we also measured internal carotid artery back pressure. We were pleased to find an extremely good correlation. Those patients who had back pressure < 25 mm Hg inevitably developed an abnormal EEG, with changes in frequency or amplitude of wave form in the affected hemisphere. Those patients in whom the back pressure was > 25 mm Hg continued to have a normal EEG pattern. In the patients in whom operation was performed with temporary clamping, based upon back pressure criteria as well as a normal EEG, there were no neurologic deficits. In our hands, the EEG appeared to be well validated based upon back pressure criteria (1). This provided a good justification for the continued use of back pressure. However, there was one additional observation that was made during this correlation. We noted that, in contrast to EEG monitoring, measurement of back pressure represented a one-time observation. Studies that examined back pressure serially during operation have demonstrated pressure variability with pressures at times dopping below a critical threshold (3). EEG, on the other hand, provided a means of continuous rather than one-time monitoring. In addition, the use of EEG monitoring eliminated the need for the additional step of making the measurement of back pressure, and therefore from the surgeon's perspective, simplified the operation. Because there was such a good correlation between EEG and back pressure, we have subsequently stopped using internal carotid artery back pressure in our institution and have gone exclusively to EEG monitoring. This was done because of the convenience in using EEG as well as the recognition of the value of continuous rather than one-time monitoring. However, because of good correlation between back pressure and EEG in our center, we can recommend the use of back pressure to those surgeons who do not have access to EEG instrumentation.

Several clinics continue to use internal carotid artery back pressure as their means of determining shunt requirement. In particular, Archie continues to make important observations as well as modifications of the back pressure method. Most recently, he described a means of measuring cerebral perfusion pressure by documenting internal carotid artery back pressure as well as jugular vein pressure. When he subtracted the jugular vein pressure from the back pressure, he noted that patients who had a cerebral perfusion pressure in excess of 18 mm Hg or an absolute internal carotid artery back pressure in excess of 25 mm Hg could safely undergo carotid endarterectomy without a shunt (2).

Summary

Internal carotid artery back pressure continues to be a reliable, well-documented method to determine collateral cerebral perfusion pressure and cerebral blood flow. Patients undergoing carotid endarterectomy for asymptomatic carotid stenosis or transient cerebral ischemia can safely undergo endarterectomy without a shunt if their internal carotid artery back pressure is in excess of 25 mm Hg. Patients with back pressures < 25 mm Hg, or those patients in whom the indication for operation is prior ipsilateral stroke, are most safely operated upon with the use of an internal shunt.

It is important to recognize that back pressure measurement is an effective means of determining collateral cerebral blood flow when deciding whether or not a temporary shunt will be required. It is no guarantee against neurologic complication related to technical problems at the endarterectomy site such as embolization during mobilization, end point problems, platelet aggregation on the intimectomized surface, or thrombosis of the reconstruction. It does provide a simple, safe, and inexpensive means for identifying the small percentage of patients who require a shunt and eliminating the need for shunting in the majority of patients undergoing carotid endarterectomy.

References

1. Ahn SS, Jordan SE, Nuwer MR, Marcus DR, Moore WS (1988) Computed electroencephalographic topographic brain mapping – A new and accurate monitor of cerebral circulation and function for patients having carotid endarterectomy. J Vasc Surg 8: 247–254
2. Archie JP Jr (1991) Technique and clinical results of carotid stump back-pressure to determine selective shunting during carotid endarterectomy. J Vasc Surg 13: 319–326
3. Beebe HG, Starr C, Slack D (1989) Carotid artery stump pressure: Its variability when measured serially. J Cardiovasc Surg 30: 19–23
4. Gnanadev DA, Wang N, Comunale FL, Reile DA (1989) Carotid artery stump pressure: How reliable is it in predicting the need for a shunt? Ann Vasc Surg 3: 313–317
5. Hays RF, Levinson SA, Wylie EJ (1972) Intraoperative measurement of carotid back pressure as a guide to operative management for carotid endarterectomy. Surgery 72: 953–960
6. Hertzer NR, Beven EG, Greenstreet RL, Humphries AS (1978) Internal carotid back pressure, intra-operative shunting, ulcerated atheroma, and the incidence of stroke during carotid endarterectomy. Surgery 83: 306–312
7. Hobson RW II, Wright CB, Sublett JW, Fedde CW, Rich NM (1974) Carotid artery back pressure and endarterectomy under regional anesthesia. Arch Surg 109: 682–687
8. Hunter GC, Sieffert G, Malone JM, Moore WS (1982) The accuracy of carotid artery back pressure as an index for shunt requirements – A reappraisal. Stroke 13: 319–326
9. Kelly JJ, Callow AD, O'Donnell TF et al. (1979) Failure of carotid stump pressures. Arch Surg 114: 1361–1366
10. McFarland HR, Pinkerton JA Jr, Frye D (1988) Continuous electroencephalographic monitoring during carotid endarterectomy. J Cardiovasc Surg 29: 12–18
11. Moore WS, Hall AD (1969) Carotid artery back pressure – A test of cerebral tolerance to temperary carotid occlusion. Arch Surg 99: 702–710
12. Moore WS, Yee JM, Hall AD (1973) Collateral cerebral blood pressure – An index of tolerance to temporary carotid occlusion. Arch Surg 106: 520–523
13. Riles TS, Imparato AM, Jacobowitz GR, Lamparello PG et al. (1994) The cause of perioperative stroke after carotid endarterectomy. J Vasc Surg 19: 206–214
14. Smith LL, Jacobson JG, Hinshaw DB (1976) Correlation of neurologic complications in pressure measurements during carotid endarterectomy. SG&O 143: 233–236

Author's address:
W. S. Moore, MD
Professor of Surgery
Chief, Section of Vascular Surgery
UCLA Center for the Health Sciences
10833 LeConte Ave., Room 72-215
Los Angeles, CA 90095-6904

Measurement of regional cerebral oxygen saturation

M. Holzschuh, C. Woertgen, A. Brawanski

Department of Neurosurgery, University of Regensburg, Regensburg, Germany

Introduction

The brain with its comparatively high metabolism is extremely sensitive to hypoxia and ischaemia. Hypoxic brain damage may occur in the case of a mismatch of oxygen supply and demand. For example, excessive demand can be found during cerebral fits. On the other hand a reduction of cerebral blood flow may lead to an inadequate delivery of oxygen. A reduction of cerebral blood flow may be caused by severe hypotension, brain oedema or vascular obstruction. Reduced cerebral blood flow leads either to a reversible loss of neural function or irreversible death of brain cells (2, 3). The degree of neurological recovery ranges from a persistent vegetative state to minor disturbances with apparent normality.

However, the measurement of cerebral blood flow is complicated and highly sophisticated technical equipment is necessary. Additionally, the current methods do not allow on-line measurement of cerebral blood flow, which is why real monitoring is not possible.

Three different monitoring methods of cerebral oxygenation were developed within the last few years: jugular bulb oximetry; tissue PO_2 monitoring; and near infrared spectroscopy. Jugular bulb oximetry was introduced into clinical practice in the mid-1980s. The oxygen saturation of the venous cerebral blood can be measured with a small catheter which is introduced into the jugular bulb. This method allows a global estimation of the oxygen extraction of the brain. The oxygen extraction depends on cerebral blood flow and cerebral oxygen metabolism (1, 4–8, 18, 19).

Another method is the tissue PO_2 monitoring. This method uses a very small electrode which is introduced through a burr hole into the white matter of the brain. This electrode measures the oxygen pressure of the brain which is a very sensitive parameter for ischaemia (10, 11, 15). Both methods – jugular bulb oximetry and tissue PO_2 monitoring – are valuable methods, but both methods are more or less invasive and bear the risk of catheter related complications. Therefore these methods are mainly used in the intensive care unit for long-term monitoring of patients with severe brain trauma.

Method of near infrared monitoring

The method of cerebral near infrared monitoring was introduced by Frans Jöbsis in 1977 (14). The in vivo near infrared spectroscopy is based on the fact that light with a wavelength between 650 and 1100 nm is able to penetrate the human skull and brain for several centimetres. There exist three light absorbing substances with a characteristic light absorbing spectrum: deoxyhaemoglobin; oxyhaemoglobin; and cytochrome a. Each of these molecules has a specific infrared absorption spectrum. The law of Lambert-Beer describing the relationship between light absorption and concentration of a certain substance is given by the following equation:

$$\log (l_0/l) = a \cdot c \cdot l = OD$$

where lo is intensity of incident light, l is intensity of transmitted light, a is extinction coefficient, c is concentration, l is path length, and OD is optical density. A change of the concentration leads to a change of the intensity of the transmitted light. With this equation the concentration of a certain substance can be calculated (9, 16).

In the Department of Neurosurgery of the University of Regensburg we used the INVOS 3100 device manufactured by Somanetics (Troy, Mich., USA). This device uses a self-adhesive sensor which consists of one light source and two light sensors (Fig. 1). Due to the two light sensors and a computer algorithm the device is able to discriminate between the superficial compartment composed of skin, galea and bone and the deep cerebral department (Fig. 2). The values are given in per cent as regional oxygen saturation. The signal represents mainly the venous compartment of the cerebral tissue (17). A decrease of the oxygen saturation value represents a decrease of cerebral blood flow or an increase of metabolism. Under stable conditions either in the operating room or during intensive care treatment we can expect a stable brain metabolism. Thus a decrease of oxygen saturation indicates a decrease of cerebral blood flow.

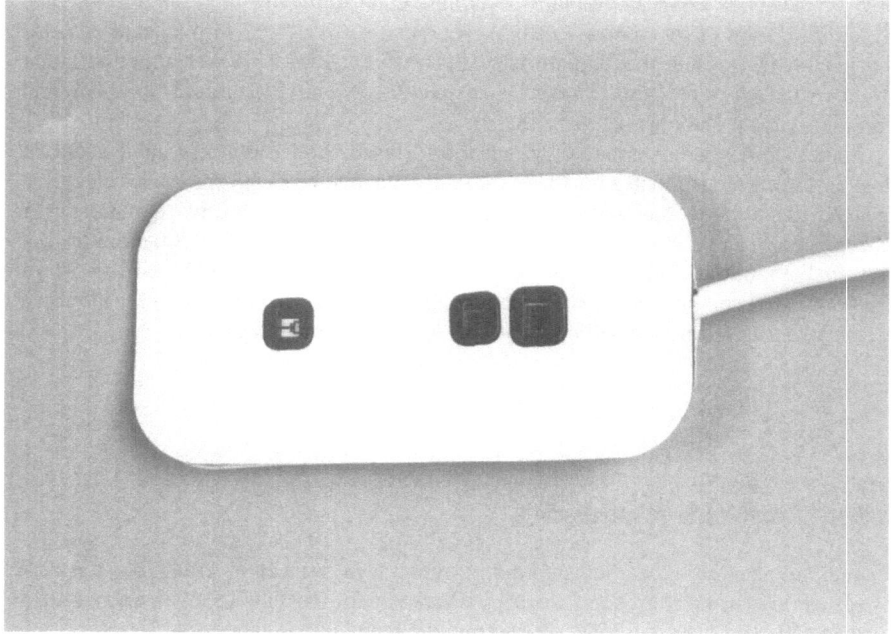

Fig. 1. Sensor of the INVOS 3100 near infrared monitor. The light source is visible on the left side, the two light sensors on the right side

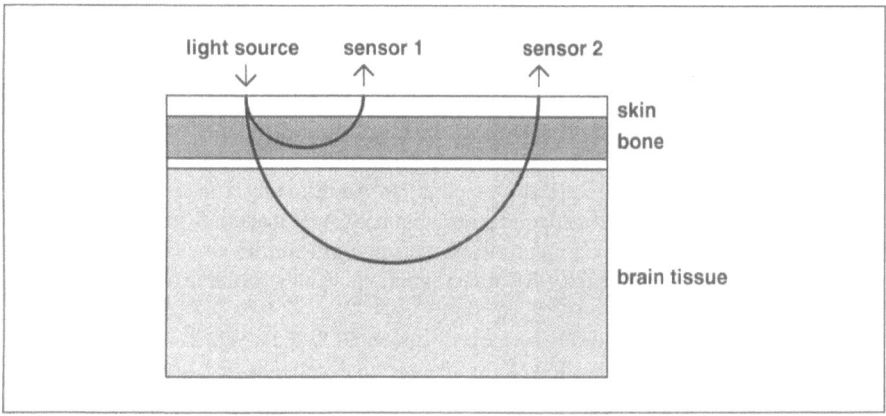

Fig. 2. Schematic representation of the mean path of the photons from the light source to the two sensors. The mean path of the photons to sensor 1 represents mainly the light from skin and bone, and that to sensor 2 mainly the light that has travelled through the cerebral tissue. The algorithm of the INVOS device uses the signal of sensor 1 as a correction of the deep signal in order to eliminate the superficial contamination

Near infrared in healthy volunteers

In a series of 50 healthy volunteers we studied the regional oxygen saturation over both frontal areas. We found an overall mean value of 70 % over the frontal areas. Additionally, we were not able to find a significant difference between different age groups (Fig. 3) (12).

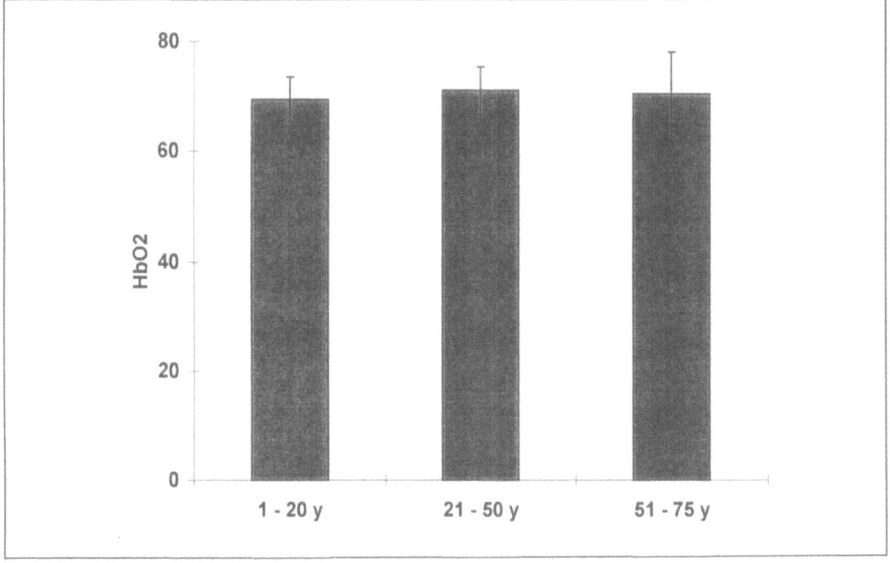

Fig. 3. Cerebral near infrared monitoring: in the group of the 50 healthy volunteers there was no significant difference of oxygen saturation (HbO$_2$) between the three age groups

Near infrared and cerebral blood flow

In a next step we wanted to find out whether an increase of cerebral blood flow without change of metabolism could be detected with the near infrared method. In 21 patients with various cerebrovascular diseases we routinely performed a cerebral blood flow (CBF) measurement with the Xenon inhalation technique. Additionally, a second study was followed after injection of 1 g acetazolamide intravenously. Acetazolamide increases cerebral blood flow without influence on metabolism. During both studies a near infrared sensor was placed on the forehead near a CBF detector and the values obtained were recorded on floppy disc.

In 18 patients we observed an increase of about 30 % of cerebral blood flow after acetazolamide. Three patients showed an inverse steal reaction due to their pathology. The near infrared results were similar. In 19 patients the saturation increased about 4.7 %. In 2 patients with inverse CBF reaction, near infrared also showed an inverse reaction. Only 1 patient showed a marked discrepancy with a decrease of CBF and an increase of saturation. From these values we calculated a positive correlation between the change of CBF and the change of saturation (Fig. 4). The absolute values, however did not correlate. Out of these results we conclude that with the near infrared method we can detect changes of cerebral blood flow after stimulation with acetazolamide. It is possible that near infrared might be useful as a screening method in order to detect a reduced reserve capacity in patients with cerebrovascular diseases.

Near infrared and tissue PO$_2$ monitoring

With the aim to evaluate the near infrared method, we studied the correlation of the near infrared results with the values of the tissue PO$_2$ monitoring method in patients with severe

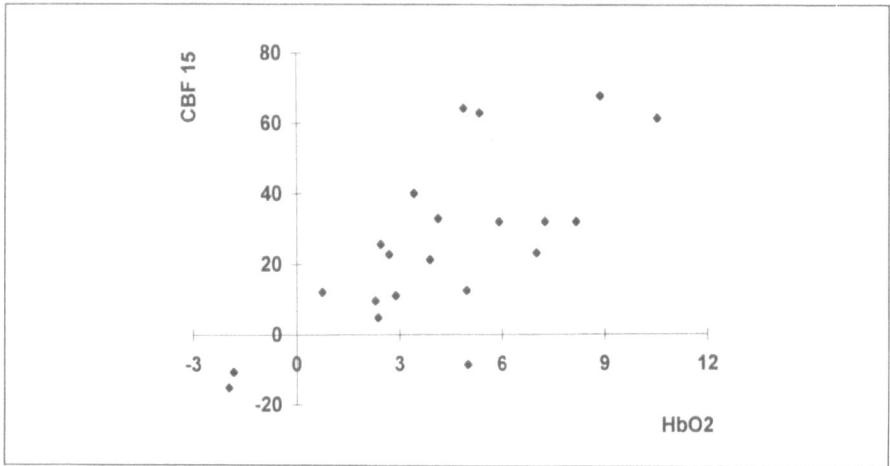

Fig. 4. Correlation between the change of cerebral blood flow (CBF 15) and the change of HbO$_2$ after stimulation with acetazolamide (r = 0.71)

head injury. As described above, tissue PO_2 measurement is an invasive method of monitoring the oxygen pressure in the white substance of the brain. Therefore a small catheter is introduced into the brain through a burr hole, in most cases together with an intracranial pressure monitoring device. The values are given in mm mercury.

We studied 10 patients with severe traumatic brain injury and parallel recording of ti-PO_2 and near infrared monitoring. We defined 137 so-called events, which means a change of > 10 % in ti-PO_2 with a duration of > 3 min. We found 79 events with a decrease of ti-PO_2 and 58 increases. In 77 % of all events we found a corresponding change in near infrared, and in 22 % there was no correlation. We calculated a positive overall correlation of the ti-PO_2 values and the near infrared values of 0.73 (Fig. 5). In 7 patients there was a strong correlation and in 3 patients we found a very poor correlation. The reason for this poor correlation might be poor signal quality due to local laceration and swelling of the skin and galea (13).

Conclusion

From these data we can conclude that the near infrared method is a non-invasive monitoring method with easy handling. The installation of the sensor and optimal placement takes about 10 min. There seems to be a good correlation of near infrared changes compared to established methods like cerebral blood flow measurement and tissue PO_2 monitoring. However, a defined threshold value of the lower saturation limit where permanent ischaemic brain damage can be expected is not yet established.

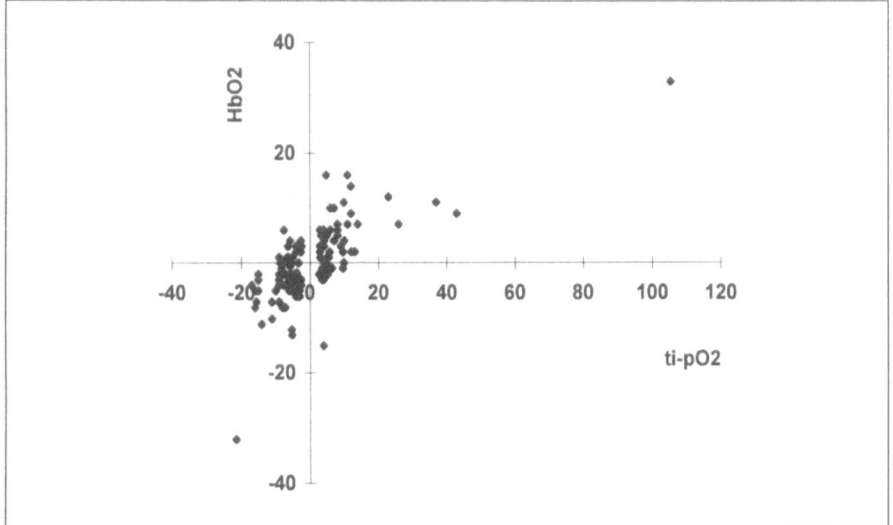

Fig. 5. Correlation between ti-PO_2 and HbO_2 in 10 patients with head injury (r = 0.73)

References

1. Andrews PJD, Dearden NM, Miller JD (1991) Jugular bulb cannulation: description of a cannulation technique and validation of a new continuous monitor. Br J Anaesth 67: 553–558
2. Avery SF, Crockard HA, Ross Russull RW (1984) Evolution and resolution of oedema following severe temporary cerebral ischaemia in the gerbil. J Neurosurg Psych 47: 604–610
3. Branston NM, Symon L, Crockard HA, Pasztor E (1974) Relationship between the cortical evoked potentials and local cortical blood flow following acute middle cerebral artery occlusion in the baboon. Exp Neurol 45: 195–208
4. Chan KH, Miller JD, Dearden NM, Andrews PJD, Midgley S (1992) The effect of changes in cerebral perfusion pressure upon middle cerebral artery blood flow velocity and jugular bulb venous oxygen saturation after severe brain injury. J Neurosurg 77: 55–61
5. Cruz J (1988) Continuous versus serial global cerebral hemometabolic monitoring. Application in acute brain trauma. Acta Neurochir Wien (Suppl) 42: 35–39
6. Cruz J, Allen SJ, Miner ME (1985) Hypoxic insults in acute brain injury. Crit Care Med 4: 284
7. Cruz J, Miner ME, Allen SJ, Alves WM, Gennarelli TA (1990) Continuous monitoring of cerebral oxygenation in acute brain injury: injection of mannitol during hyperventilation. J Neurosurg 73: 725–730
8. Dearden NM (1991) Jugular bulb venous oxygen saturation in the management of severe head injury. Curr Opin Anaesth 4: 279–286
9. Fahnenstich H (1993) Nahinfrarotspektroskopie – eine neue Methode zum nicht invasiven Monitoring zerebraler Hämodynamik. Klin Pädiatr 205: 398–403
10. Fleckenstein W, Maas AIR, Nollert G, de Jong DA (1990) Oxygen pressure in cerebrospinal fluid. In: Ehrly AM, et al. (eds.) Clinical oxygen pressure measurement, vol 2. Blackwell Ueberreuter, Berlin, pp 368–395
11. Fleckenstein W, Nowak G, Kehler U, Maas AIR, Dellbrügge HJ, de Jong DA, Hess M, Nollert G (1990) Oxygen pressure measurements in cerebrospinal fluid. Med Tech 110: 44–53
12. Holzschuh M, Brawanski A, Kropf M (1994) First experience with near-infrared cerebral oximetry in head injury. Stroke 25: 757
13. Holzschuh M, Woertgen C, Metz C, Brawanski A (1996) Dynamic changes of cerebral oxygenation measured by brain tissue oxygen pressure and near infrared spectroscopy. Neurol Res, in press
14. Jöbsis FF (1977) Noninvasive, infrared monitoring of cerebral and myocardial oxygen sufficiency and circulatory parameters. Science 198: 1264–1267
15. Maas AIR, Fleckenstein W, de Jong DA, van Santbrink H (1993) Monitoring cerebral oxygenation: experimental studies and preliminary clinical results of continuous monitoring of cerebrospinal fluid and brain tissue oxygen tension. Acta Neurochir (Suppl) 59: 50–57
16. McCormick PW, Stewart M, Goetting MG, Dujovny M, Lewis G, Ausman JI (1991) Noninvasive cerebral optical spectroscopy for monitoring cerebral oxygen delivery and hemodynamics. Crit Care Med 19: 89–97
17. McCormick PW, Stewart M, Lewis G (1991) Noninvasive measurement of regional cerebrovascular oxygen saturation in humans using optical spectroscopy. SPIE 1431: 294–302
18. Robertson CS, Contant CF, Gokaslan ZL, Narayan RK, Grossman RG (1992) Cerebral blood flow, arteriovenous oxygen difference and outcome in head injured patients. J Neurol Neurosurg Psychiat 55: 594–603
19. Sheinberg M, Kanter MJ, Robertson CS, Contant CF, Narayan RK, Grossman RG (1992) Continuous monitoring of jugular venous oxygen saturation in head-injured patients. J Neurosurg 76: 212–217

Author's address:
M. Holzschuh, M.D.
Neurochirurgische Universitätsklinik Regensburg
Franz-Josef-Strauß-Allee 11
93053 Regensburg, Germany

Postoperative evaluation of blood viscoelasticity response during carotid endarterectomy – considerable consequences for intraoperative management?

M. Hold

Department of Surgery, Hanuschkrankenhaus, Vienna, Austria

Introduction

This report of a study (16) on changes of characteristics of blood, sampled from the ipsilateral jugular vein during carotid endarterectomy may emphasize the risks of clamping of the cerebral arteries. The aim of carotid surgery is to preserve cerebral cells as much possible. Absence of neurological deficit alone is an insufficient measure of the benefit of the operation.

Increased whole blood viscosity has been observed in patients with focally reduced cerebral blood flow (14, 22, 26). Whole blood is a non-Newtonian liquid with viscosity depending on the shear rate applied to the liquid. The shear stress is the shearing force of adjacent layers of blood per unit area and decreases with decreasing flow rate (11). The term shear rate is almost synonymous with velocity gradient, it is directly proportional to velocity of blood flow and inversely proportional to vessel radius.

Reduction of shear rate can produce a perfusion defect in the microvessels which results in aggregation of erythrocytes and in stimulation of platelets and polymorph nuclear leucocytes (PMNL) followed by production and release of substances that causes vasoconstriction and enhanced vessel patency and further chemotaxis (3, 24). As blood flow and shear rate decrease to very low levels, complex viscosity markedly increases (31). Viscosity η' represents the energy-dissipating component, the elasticity η'' the energy-storing component of the complex viscosity of whole blood, lying between Newtonian fluid and Hooke's law characteristics. The phase interchange between both components, the phase angle Φ represents the part of elastic energy stored in the circulating blood from the total energy required to keep it in motion (Fig. 1). Other factors that determine blood viscosity include hematocrit, erythrocyte aggregation, erythrocyte flexibility, platelet aggregation, plasma viscosity and shear rate (21). Flexibility or shear resistance (dyn/cm^2) is a measure of the force which is required to detach blood cell aggregates. Shear resistance increases with decreasing erythrocyte deformability (17). The deformability is affected mostly by the viscosity of blood cell cytoplasm. Aggregation is modified by proteins (fibrinogen and globulin), the state of the cell membrane and the ionic concentration of the fluid.

Of these factors, hematocrit plays the most important role, the viscosity almost doubles at a hematocrit of 50 % compared to that at 35 % (6). Hemodynamically relevant arterial stenoses increases blood viscosity in the in-flowing organ. Responsible for this reaction are not so much changes in the metabolic process through oxygen and substrate deficit, but the decrease in velocity itself (10, 13). Besides other matters the flow characteristics of blood are dependent on the degree of thrombocytes and PMNL stimulation produced by collision, but mostly through intercellular and endothelial contact (18, 29). Flow deceleration with incurring delayed capillary passage decreases, on the one hand, collision rate,

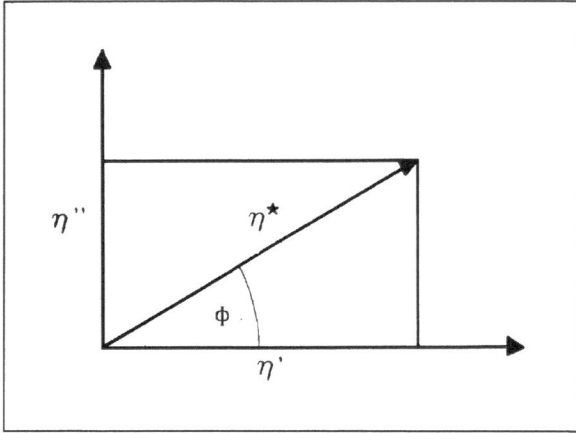

Fig. 1. Diagram of viscoelasticity parameters in Gauss's numeric level. The index of complex viscosity η^* is represented as vector, whereby the imaginary part (η") forms the y-axis and the real part (θ') the x-axis. The angle between both parts is called the phase angle Φ.

but on the other increases the contact time which is the principle stimulating factor in these cells.

Capillary response is very sensitive to even slight alteration in the microcirculatory pathophysiology. Its early reaction to ischemia is measured by blood viscosity from the ipsilateral internal jugular vein during the different phases of carotid endarterectomy. The routine use of an intraluminal shunt for cerebral protection during carotid endarterectomy has been the topic of much controversy ever since its initiation. Carotid endarterectomies are performed in our department under local anaesthesia and indwelling shunt. In almost 20 % of these cases, transient but major neurological deficits are observed at clamping, vanishing immediately, when the shunt is installed.

The well known critics against the usage of an indwelling shunt led us to study the response of clamping of the internal carotid artery during endarterectomy and blood viscoelasticity and density as an indirect parameter of the extent of ischemia. The aim is, threefold: first, to demonstrate if clamping of the carotid artery produces significant cerebral capillary endothelial and blood cell response resulting in a shift of blood viscoelasticity. Second: do these changes occur when atherosclerotic lesions are unilateral and collaterals are judged to be sufficient. Third: is this situation improved if blood flow is reiterated by shunt and following endarterectomy.

Method

During a 3-month-period, 17 patients (10 men, 7 women, mean age 66.7) undergoing carotid endarterectomy with solely unilateral pathological lesions and related ipsilateral symptomatic consented to join this study. All patients had a history of stroke with remitted neurologic symptoms. Five patients had diabetes mellitus, all were hypertensive with good response to nifedipine (Adalat, Bayer, Germany) therapy. Preoperative blood count and coagulation parameters were non pathological. The cerebral perfusion reserve was assessed by measuring the middle cerebral artery velocity with a transcranial Doppler. No difference was noticed compared to the contralateral side. Patients with bilateral carotid involvement or neoplastic disease were excluded.

During the operation blood pressure was kept at 20 % over the baseline value but no less than 150 mm Hg. After careful preparation of the carotid bifurcation, a Drum Cartridge catheter with 1.1 mm bore was installed into the internal jugular vein 5 cm cephalad. Following the administration of 5000 IU Na-Heparin i.v., and after the first 5cc blood sample was discarded, 2 potassium-EDTA 5cc test tubes (Vacutainer) were filled and blood viscoelasticity and plasma density were measured with the oscillating capillary rheometer and densimeter (OCR-D, A. Paar KG, Graz, Austria) at 20° Celsius following the method described by Thurston and modified by Chmiel et al. (7), Kenner (19), Kratky et al. (21), Moser et al. (25).

Analysis was performed at a shear rate of 1 and 2 s^{-1}, which corresponds nearest to capillary circulation (18, 30). The plasma viscoelasticity and density values were assessed after separation of plasma by conventional centrifugation of the first tube for 5 min at 4000 g and blood viscoleasticity and density from the whole blood out of the second tube. Hematocrit was determined with a microhematocrit centrifuge. The densitometer works at a resolution of 10^{-4} g/cm. Flexibility, aggregation and shear resistance were computed on these measurements.

Further sampling and assessments were carried in the same manner throughout the operative procedure. The second sampling was drawn during clamping before insertion of the shunt, the third one 3 min after shunting, the fourth immediately preceding the patch arteriotomy closure, the fifth during reclamping so as to be able to remove the intraluminal shunt and finish the patch closure, the sixth and last sample was drawn at the end of the operation before wound closure. A standardisation of the clamping time was rejected because of ethical reasons. It ranged between 50 and 210 s. The shunting time lay between 19 and 33 min. Each patient received 500 ml Ringer solution at the onset of the operation, at approximately 20 drops/min. Each received 40 mg Dexamethason (Fortecortin, Hoechst, Germany) i.v. at the same time as 5000 U Heparin i.v., 4 min before the first blood sampling. No other medication which could influence blood viscosity were administrated pre- or intraoperatively.

In one patient the indwelling shunt was inadvertently occluded. This was noticed at the removal of the shunt, where a kinking was found. This case was excluded from statistical analysis and will be discussed separately.

Changes in venous blood viscosity were evaluated and comparative analysis performed with the baseline value measured primarily, and this at a shear rate of $\Phi = 1$, and 2 s^{-1}.

For our analysis of the three factors: phase angle, viscous and elastic component of the whole blood viscosity the deviation from the normal value of healthy individuals were computed, whereas the absolute values of shear resistance, aggregation, flexibility, blood density and density hematocrit were used. Subsequent measurements were compared to their initial values of the first samplings. Wilcoxon's log rank test for dependent variables and Student's t-test for dependent variables were used for the statistical analysis with the SAS software package (SAS-Institute Inc. Gary, N. C., USA).

Results

No perioperative neurological incidence was noticed. Patients were conscious and in constant vocal contact with the anaesthetist standing by.

As Fig. 2 shows, the deviation of viscosity, elasticity and phase angle from the normal values increases clearly after clamping to decline and almost diminish during shunt perfusion and after completion of endarterectomy. Between the first and fourth sampling, there was no significant different alteration in the viscoelastic phase angle (p = 0.1030). At shear rates of 1 - 2 s^{-1}, the difference in alteration of the deviation of the viscous component from the normal was statistically significant in the 2nd and 4th sampling (p = 0.0372, 0.0313), p of the elastic component at $\Phi = 1$ s^{-1} was 0.0605, however, at $\Phi = 2$ s^{-1} 0.0404. A biphasic curve is also present when computed flexibility, shear resistance and erythrocyte aggregation are measured (Fig 3).

A normal distribution was seen only in the measured value of aggregation, therefore the t-test for dependent variables was used and showed a statistically significant difference between the first and fourth sampling (p = 0.0366).

As depicted in Fig. 4, whole blood density (g/ml) and hematocrit specific gravity measured through plasma and blood density differentiate significantly in the first and fourth sampling (p = 0.0654, 0.0196), in the second and fourth (p = 0.0218, 0.0249) and in the fourth and fifth sampling (p = 0.0040, 0.0086). Both these parameters are determined mostly by the water content. No statistical significance was observed in plasma density and viscosity measurements throughout the course of the procedure.

Discussion

Little is known about the degree of diffuse cerebral cell destruction occurring during carotid endarterectomy. Pure permanent neurological deficits are luckily relatively rare; they are reported to be in the area of 2 to 10 % in the literature [Boontje 1994]. The aim, however, is to prevent any type of diffuse cerebral deterioration may it be clinically mute. It has been up to now the general point of view that cerebral protection during clamping of the carotid artery was needed in just a few cases, mostly for those in whom the contralateral or collateral blood flow was inadequate. In order to differentiate patients who could less tolerate carotid clamping, many well known and discussed methods of monitoring are applied. From these proceedings, it was concluded that an indwelling shunt was actually necessary in only 10 to 3 0% of cases (9, 12, 27). In this study group no intraoperative neurological incidence was noticed, although transient deficit occurs in about 20 % of our patients at clamping.

Our study demonstrates that fluid characteristics of blood deteriorates during clamping probably as a response to shear rate reduction in the capillary network. This may indicate that perfusion pressure was not compensated by collateral or contralateral blood flow although solely unilateral lesions with adequate peripheral distribution was seen in the angiogram. This is most evident in one case where the intraluminal shunt did not function due to inadvertent occlusion, which was not noticed until the shunt was removed at the end of the procedure (Fig. 5). Also in this case no neurological deficits were observed.

An increase in whole blood viscosity in presence of arteriosclerotic lesions has been substantiated by many studies (2, 8, 14, 20). Also ischemia, whether acute or chronic, has been shown to produce the same effect. Tissue perfusion is dependent among other things on the PMNL and platelet stimulation produced when colliding and, mostly through intercellular and endothelium contact (28). In the low flow state leucocyte passage through the capillary network is stopped and individual capillaries are not perfused (1, 15, 23, 32, 33).

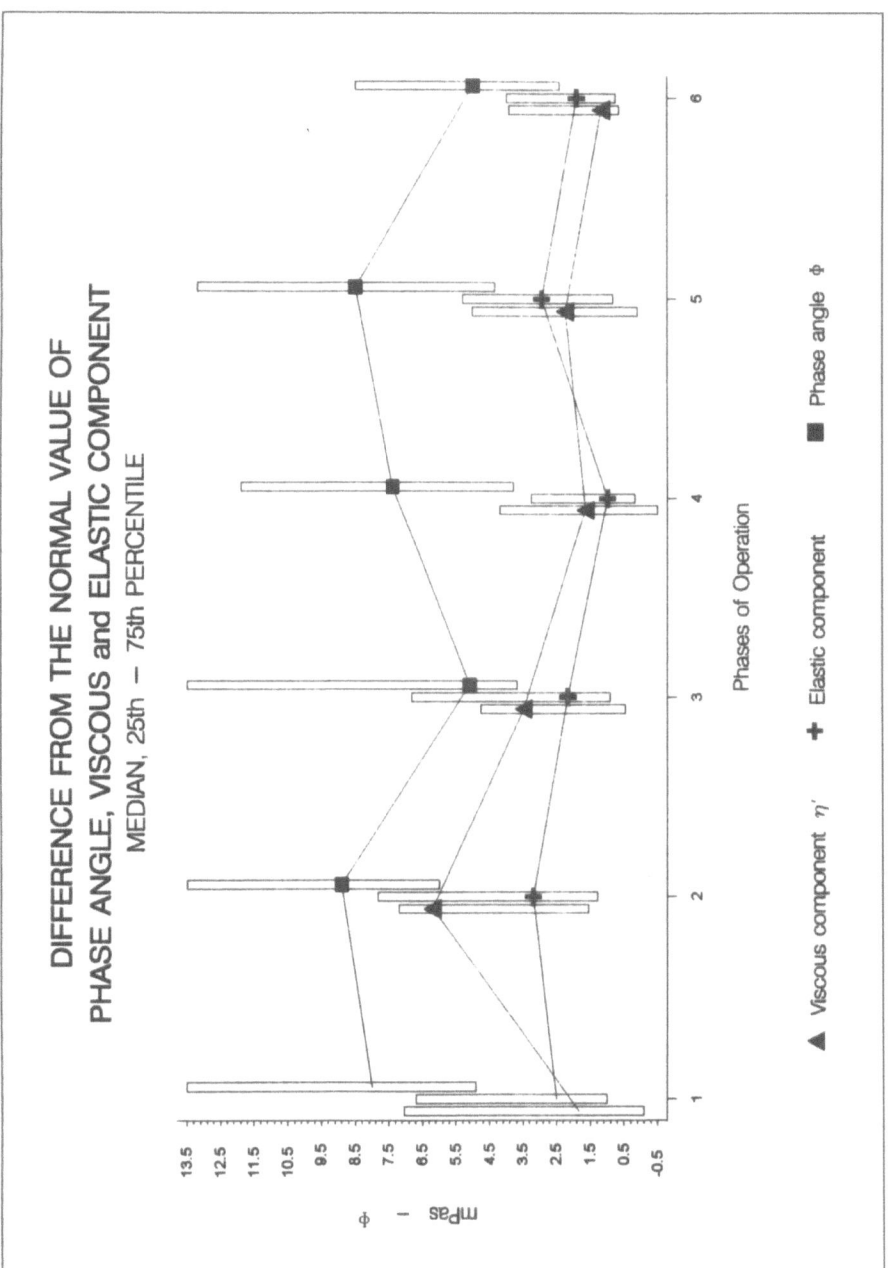

Fig. 2. The median deviation and 25th – 75th percentile of the viscous and elastic part of the complex viscosity and of the phase angle from the normal values of whole blood at a shear rate of 1 s^{-1} at the six defined phases of operation. P of the difference in alteration of the phase angle Φ at the 2nd and 4th sampling was 0.1030, of the elastic component η' 0.0605, of the viscous component 0.0372.

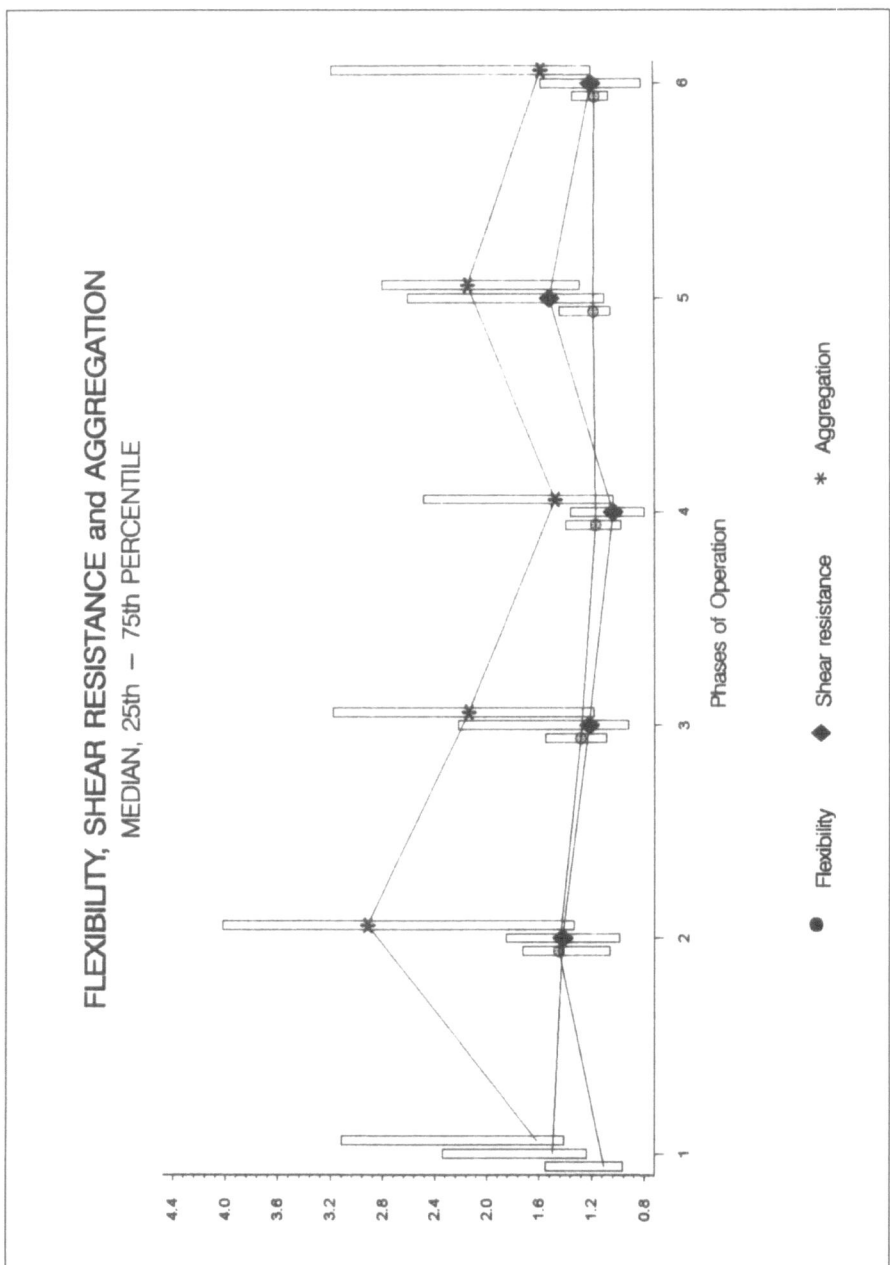

Fig. 3. The median deviation and 25th – 75th percentile of flexibility, shear resistance and aggregation at the six defined phases of operation. P of the alteration of aggregation at the 1st and 4th sampling was 0.0366.

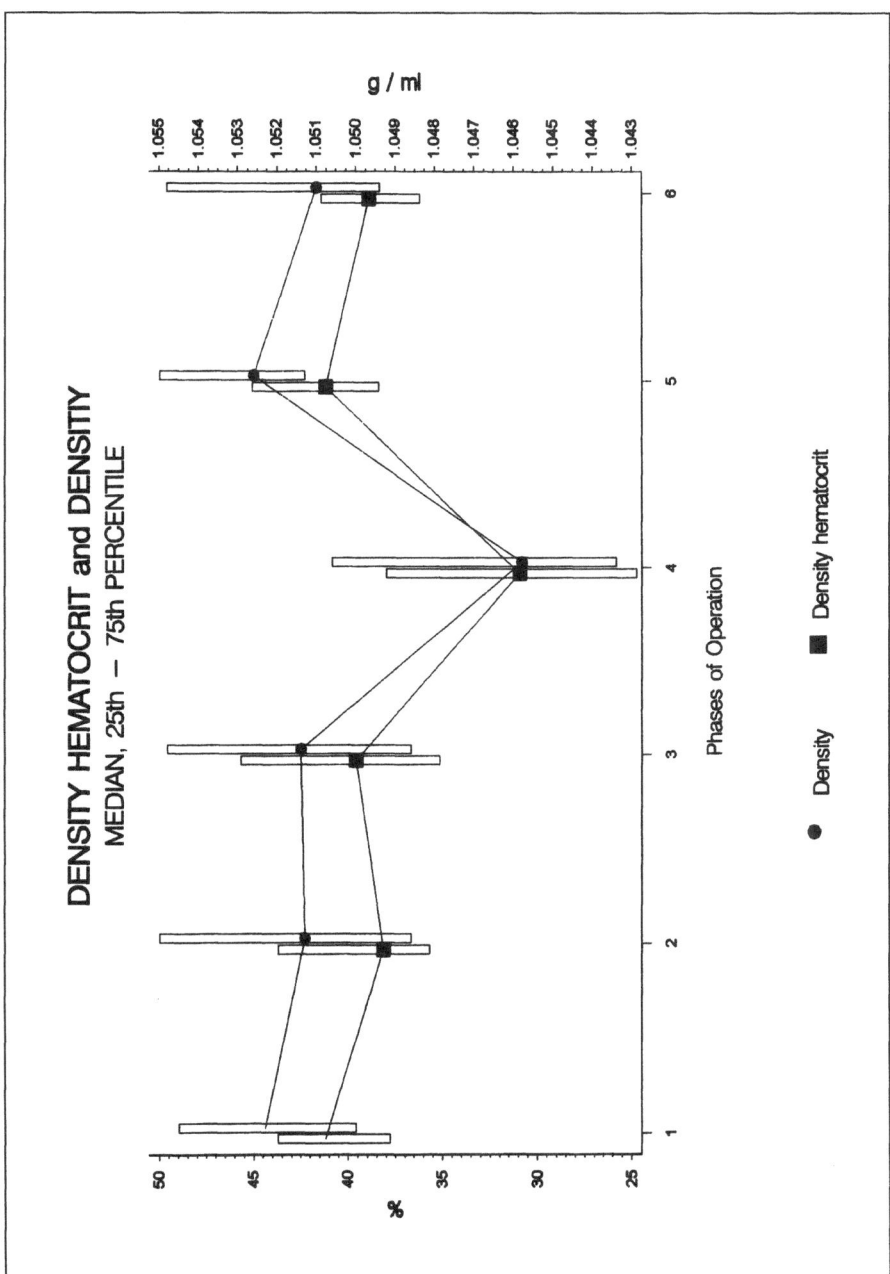

Fig. 4. Median deviation and 25th – 75th percentile of the hematocrit density and density at the six defined phases of operation. Hematocrit density and whole blood density differentiate in the 1st and 4th (p = 0.0654, 0.019869), in the 2nd and 4th (p = 0.0218, 0.0249) and in the 4th and 5th sampling (p = 0.0040, 0.0086).

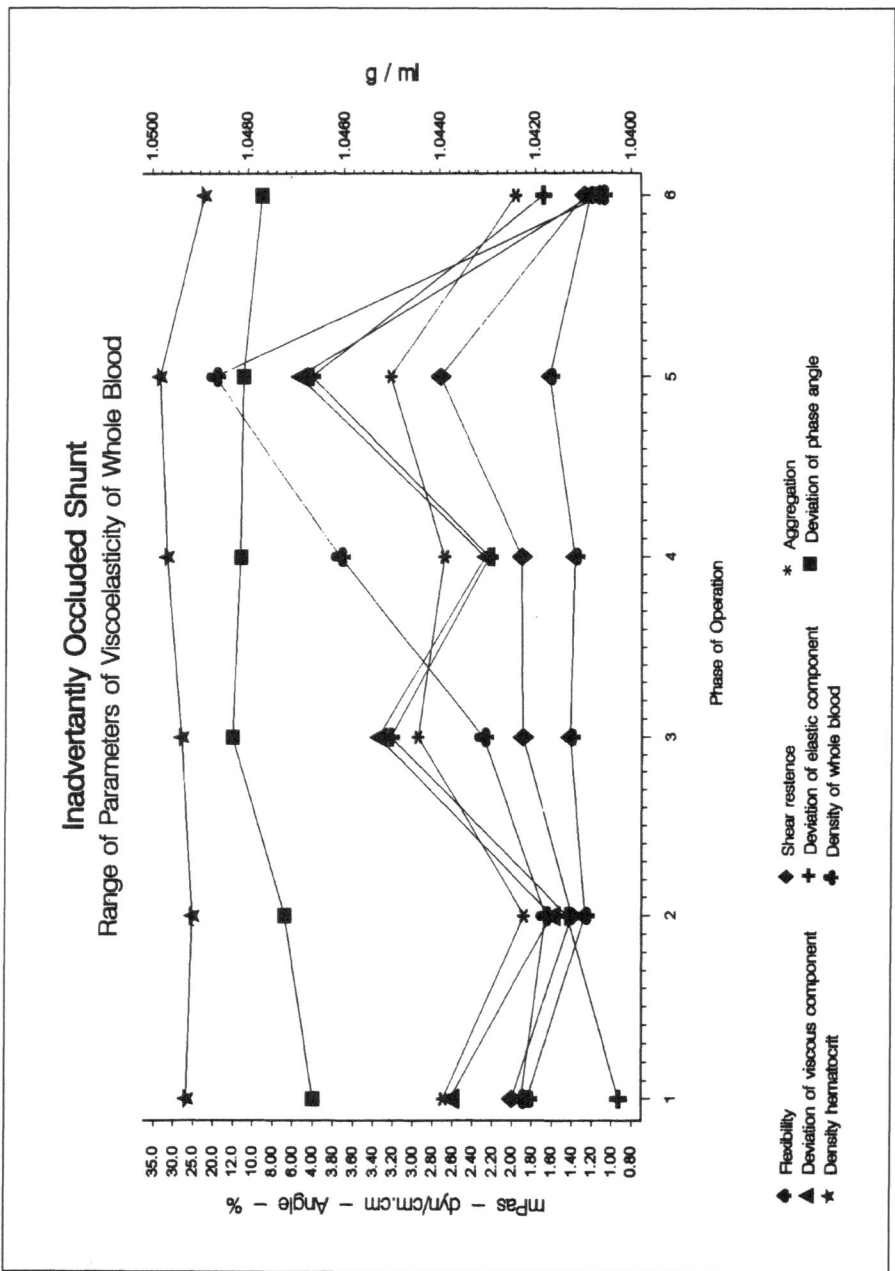

Fig. 5. Shear resistance, density, hematocrit density and deviation of the viscous and elastic part of complex viscosity and of the phase angle from the normal at a shear rate of 1 s⁻¹ at the six defined phases of operation, when the shunt was inadvertently occluded during endarterectomy procedure, following sufficient initial functioning, as demonstrated in sample 3.

Restoration of normal perfusion pressure after prolonged duration of low flow state will not enable all granulocytes to be removed from the capillaries. Granulocytes capillary plugging appears to be the microvascular origin of the non-reflow phenomenon as observed in whole organs during ischemia (1, 15, 28). This is intensified by release of lysosomal granules into tissue parenchyma in addition to local hypoxia and formation of oxygen free radicals, starting the well known cascade of lipid peroxidation (10, 23, 29).

Capillaries and venules downstream to the stenosis are probably dilated, and hence may cause a volume shift into the interstitium resulting in an increase in the venous density observed in our study. As already mentioned, the second and third sampling are not exactly definable and this explains the great variations in their values, however a general negative tendency compared to the baseline values can be observed at the second sampling as a result of flow stagnation at clamping. In contrast to this an amelioration can be seen at the third sampling, shortly after restoration of flow. This tendency continues on in the fourth sample after 19 to 33 min of shunting, exceeding the baseline values as a sign of improved perfusion.

In the fourth sampling, there is a decrease in the density and density hematocrit, possibly caused by the intravascular fluid shift as response to the increased perfusion pressure and capillary constriction. As a response to the second clamping of the carotid artery with the subsequent sudden pressure drop, capillaries react with dilation and again a fluid shift into the interstitium, as shown by the increase of density and density hematocrit. Changes in plasma density and plasma viscosity are present, but with a lower and delayed amplitude. This underscores the instantaneous blood cellular reaction in this mechanism.

These reactions are reversible, however, when an intraluminal shunt is installed, hence we tend to favour this form of cerebral protection for carotid endarterectomy although some authors believe that the possible complications may exceed the benefit derived from its use.

This investigation shows that it is possible to measure with the capillary rheometer and densimeter, beside whole blood density, the viscous and elastic part of complex viscosity and from this the shear resistance of circulating blood at different, mostly at a low-flow state of velocity as exists in the capillary network. An increase in whole blood viscosity is observed following carotid clamping which may be the result of cell aggregation more than perfusion drop alone. As the viscosity curve shows, sufficient restoration of shear velocity while shunting and after repair causes not only an improvement but exceeds the baseline values. This proves the positive effect of undisturbed flow while shunting and following repair.

Although clinically relevant transient neurological deficits have a relative low incidence, cerebral protection at the level of microcirculation may be more important than previously thought. As demonstrated in this study, clamping of the carotid artery does produce a shift in the fluid characteristics probably through cerebral capillary endothelial and blood cell response although lesions are unilateral and collateral blood perfusion is judged to be sufficient in the angiogram. Which raises the question whether these changes of fluid characteristics correlate with destruction of cerebral cells and if usual monitoring systems are able to detect these distinct processes.

References

1. Ames A, Wright RL, Kowada M, Thurston JM, Majno G (1986) Cerebral ischemia. II. The no-reflow phenomenon. Am J Pathol 52: 437–453
2. Anadere I, Chmiel H, Hess H, Thurston GB (1979) Clinical blood rheology. Biorheol 16: 171–178
3. Bagge U, Bränemark P-I (1979) White blood cell rheology. Adv Microcirc, 1–17
4. Boontje AH (1994) Carotid endarterectomy without a temporary indwelling shunt: results and analysis of back pressure measurements. Cardiovasc Surg 2 (5): 549–554
5. Callow AD (1989) Cerbrovascular insufficiency. In Haimovici H (eds): Vascular Surgery, Principles and Techniques, Norwalk, Appleton-Lange pp 719–749
6. Charara J, Aurengo A, Lelievre JC, Lacombe C (1985) Quantitative characterization of blood rheological behavior in transient flow with a modelincluding a structure parameter. Biorheology 22 (6): 509–520
7. Chmiel H, Schweizer P, Krause K-H, Framing W (1976) New methods of measuring the different rheological parameters in blood. Microcirculation 1: 171–178
8. Craveri A, Tornaghi G, Paganardi L, Di Bella M, Gallo E, Stanzani M (1987) Aumento della viscosita eritrocitaria e plasmatica in pazienti affetti da vasculopatia aterosclerotica a diversa localizzazione. Minerva Med 78 (12): 815–22
9. D'Addato M, Pedrinie L, Vitacchiano G (1993) Intraoperative cerebral monitoring in carotid surgery Europ J Vasc Surg 7 (Suppl A): 16–20
10. Dahinden CA, Fehr J, Hugli TE (1983) Role of cell surface contact in the kinetics of superoxide production by granulocytes. J Clin Invest 72 (1): 113–121
11. Dormandy JA (1970) Clinical significance of blood viscosity, Hunterien Lecture, Annals of the Royal College of Surgeons of England 47: 211–228
12. Fetter T, Horsch S, Haupt WF, Ktenidis K (1995) Monitoring somatosensory evoked potentials during carotid endarterectomy. Orvosi Hetilap, 136 (41): 2221–3
13. Gaehtgens P, Ley K, Pries, AR, Müller R (1985) Wechselwirkung zwischen Leukozyten und Blutströmung in der Mikrozirkulation Entzündung u. Rheologie der Leukozyten. Basel, Karger, pp 16–30
14. Grotta J, Ackerman R, Correia J, Fallick G, Chang J (1982) Whole blood viscosity parameters and cerebral blood flow. Stroke 13: 296–301
15. Hallenbeck JM, Dutka AJ, Tanishima T, Kochanek PM, Kumaroo KK, Thompson CB, Obrenovitch TP, Contreras TJ (1986) Polymorphonuclear leukocyte accumulation in brain regions with low blood flow during the early postischemic period. Stroke 17: 246–253
16. Hold M, Merrelaar JJ, Hollaus P, Bull PG, Denck H (1992) Blood viscoelasticity response during carotid endarterectomy. J Cerebr Blood F Met 12: 326–333
17. Johnson G Jr, Keagy BA (1985) Viscous factors in peripheral tissue perfusion. J Vasc Surg 2: 530
18. Kenner T (1982) Physiological measurement in circulation research. Med Progr Technol 9: 67–74
19. Kenner T, Leopold H, Hinghofer-Szalkay H (1977) Kontinuierliche Präzisionsmessung der Dichte des arteriellen Blutes. Wr med Wochenschr 127: 19–21
20. Koppensteiner R, Graninger W, Minar E, Kretschmer G, Ehringer H (1988) Haemorheologie und Akute Phase Reaktion nach Thrombendarteriektomie der extracraniellen Arteria carotis. Klin Wochenschr 66 (9): 379–384
21. Kratky O, Leopold H, Stabinger H (1973) The determination of the partial specific volume of proteins by the mechanical oscillator technique, In Hirs CHW and Timasheff SN (eds): Methods in Enzymology. New York, Academic Press, pp 98–110
22. Lechner H, Niederkorn K, Suzuki H (1987) Hemorheologic parameters in correlation to extracranial carotid artery disease in patients with acute cerebrovascular disorders. Eur Neurol, 27 (3): 139–141
23. Levis DH (1984) The response of the microvasculature in skeletal muscle to hemorrhage, trauma and ischemia. Prog appl Microcirc 5: 127–138
24. Litwin MS, Chapman K (1970) Physical factors affecting human blood viscosity. J Surg Res 10: 433
25. Moser M, Hinghofer-Szalkay H, Kenner Th, Holzer, H (1980) Die Bestimmung des kolloidosmotischen Drucks aus der Plasmadichte mittels der Biegerschwingermethode. J Clin Chem Clin Biochem 18: 233–236
26. Ott EO, Lechner H, Aranibar A (1974) High blood viscosity syndrom in cerebral infarction. Stroke 5: 330–333
27. Palombo D, Porta C, Peinetti F, Brustia P, Udini M, Antico A, Cantallupi D, Varetto T (1994) Cerebral reserve and indications for shunting in carotid surgery. Cardiovascular Surgery, 2 (1): 32–6 Seite: 18
28. Schmid-Schönbein GW (1987) Capillary plugging by granulocytes and the no-reflow phenomenon in the microcirculation. Fed Proc 46 (7): 2397–2401
29. Schmid-Schönbein GW, Usami S, Skalak R, Chien S (1980) The interaction of leukocytes and erythrocytes in capillary and postcapillary vessels. Microvascular Research 19: 45–70
30. Schneditz D, Rainer F, Kenner T (1987) Viscoelastic properties of whole blood. Influence of fast sedimenting red blood cell aggregates. Biorheology 24: 13–22

31. Sakuta S (1981) Blood filtrability in cerebrovascular disorders, with special reference to erythrocyte defor-mability and ATP content. Stroke 12: 6; 824–828
32. Skalak R (1984) Aggregation and disaggregation of red blood cells. Biorheology 21 (4): 463–476
33. Skalak R, Branemark P-I (1969) Deformation of red blood cells in capillaries. Science 164: 717–719
34. Thurston GB (1972) Viscoelasticity of human blood. J Biophys 12: 1205–1217
35. Thurston GB (1979) Rheological parameters for the viscosity, viscoelasticity and thixotropy of blood. Biorheol 16: 149–162
36. Walitza E, Anadere I, Chmiel H, Witte S (1988) Evaluation of viscoelasticity measurements of human blood. Biorheol 25 (1-2): 209–217

Author's address:
M. Hold, M.D.
Department of Surgery
Hanuschkrankenhaus
Heinrich-Collin-Str. 30
1140 Vienna, Austria

Scintigraphic methods (PET, SPECT) to assess disturbances of the cerebral function before and after carotid endarterectomy (CEA)

M. Grond

Max-Planck-Institut für Neurologische Forschung, Cologne, Germany

Stenosis or occlusion of the internal carotid artery is one of the major aetiological factors leading to infarction. According to the NINCDS Stroke Data Bank (14) stroke cases can be classified into the following subgroups: 8.9 % of infarctions are due to large artery atherosclerosis, 5.4 % are infarctions with tandem arterial pathology where an extracranial lesion is insufficient in itself to account for stroke on haemodynamic grounds but possibly serves as an embolic source.

There is only inconsistent correlation between the degree of carotid stenosis and haemodynamic status of the ipsilateral cerebral circulation. The collateral circulatory pathways are of great importance and since collateral circulation is variable, there is no critical degree of carotid stenosis that consistently produces haemodynamic compromise of the cerebral circulation. Therefore, cerebral haemodynamics have to be investigated more closely in this complex multifactorial disease in order to determine its importance. Advances in noninvasive techniques have made it possible to evaluate regional cerebral haemodynamics in individual patients.

Positron Emission Tomography (PET) of the brain provides quantitative maps of several important physiological variables including cerebral blood flow (CBF), cerebral blood volume (CBV), cerebral metabolic rate of oxygen metabolism ($CMRO_2$) and of glucose metabolism (CMR-GLU). These variables can be measured noninvasively and repeatedly in stroke patients. Additional variables such as oxygen extraction fraction (OEF) and glucose extraction fraction (GEF) can be derived from these data. What we are looking for is haemodynamic inadequacy caused by carotid stenosis and which implies brain blood flow mismatched to local metabolic demand.

Besides cerebrovascular resistance regional cerebral perfusion pressure is the crucial haemodynamic factor (13). Local arterial occlusive disease can produce corresponding reductions in perfusion pressure. Patients with arterial occlusive disease are protected against ischaemic episodes to a certain point by compensatory mechanisms which help to prevent ischaemia when perfusion pressure drops. This condition, studied by PET (6) in patients with uni- or bilateral carotid artery disease is indicated by regional vasodilation manifest as a focal increase in CBV in the supply territory of the occluded artery. The ratio of CBF to CBV is an indicator of local perfusion pressure and therefore a measure of the perfusion reserve. When the perfusion reserve is exhausted at maximal vasodilation, any further decrease in arterial input pressure produces a proportional decrease in both CBF and the CBF/CBV ratio. In this condition of haemodynamic decompensation, the brain must draw on the oxygen carriage reserve to prevent energy failure and loss of function, as evidenced by an increase of OEF from the normal 40–50 % up to 85 %.

This haemodynamic situation is called misery perfusion (1) and can be found in 10 to 15 % of patients with cervical occlusive disease (6). As we know from our own series of 8 patients with severe unilateral carotid stenosis studied with multitracer PET there were focal changes in every patient upon visual examination either in CBF, CBV, GEF and/or OEF (5).

The pathological findings that can be assessed with PET can be classified as follows:

Irreversible infarct: Oxygen metabolism or blood flow below viability threshold of 65 µmol/100 g per min or 12 ml/100 g per min, respectively (2, 12).

Misery perfusion: Oxygen metabolism above viability threshold, increased extraction fraction due to insufficient blood flow (1).

Hyperperfusion: Blood flow exceeds metabolic needs, decreased oxygen extraction fraction (10).

Anaerobic glycolysis: Increased glucose / oxygen metabolic ratio (17).

Figure 1 shows a PET study of a 50-year-old female 24 h after ischaemic stroke in the territory of the right middle cerebral artery (7). This example demonstrates the heterogeneity of changes in physiologic variables in early stroke as there is misery perfusion and anaerobic glycolysis in the borber zone of the infarct at the same time. PET images of the measured variables clearly demonstrate the flow defect on CBF image and the metabolic disturbance in CMRO$_2$ and CMR-GLU. The flow defect, however, is larger than the oxygen and glucose metabolism defect, leaving border zone regions with preserved oxygen and glucose consumption and therefore increased OEF and GEF. This anterior portion is preserved at the later CT. In the posterior rim, however, oxygen metabolism is more

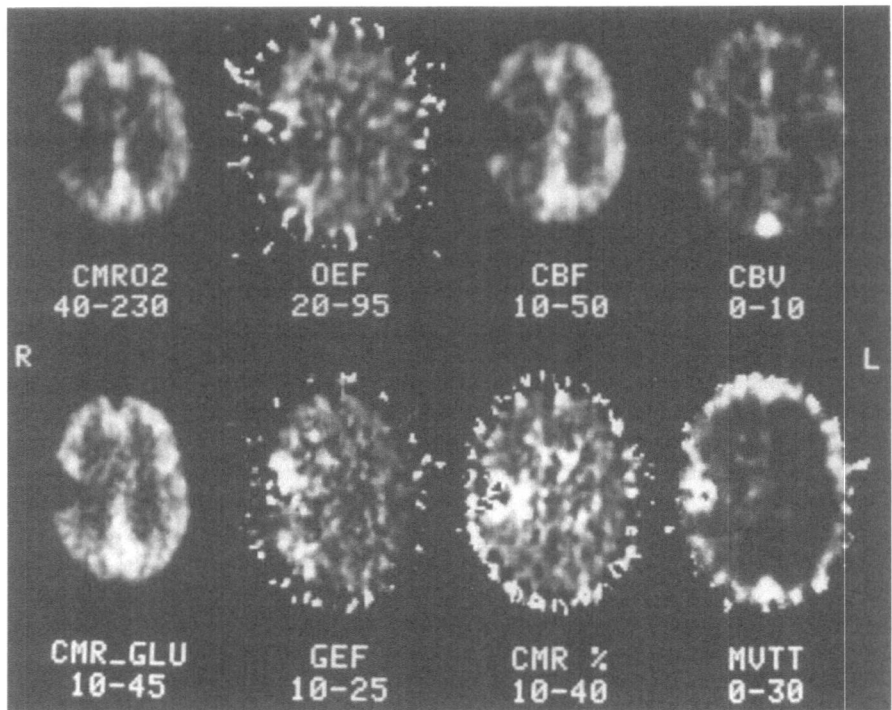

Fig. 1

severely impaired than glucose metabolism leading to an increase in the ratio of glucose to oxygen consumption (CMR %) indicative of anaerobic gycolysis. On later CT this area is infarcted.

We know from the pathophysiological considerations given before, that the areas with misery perfusion are those that are especially vulnerable to reduction in cerebral perfusion pressure and have a tendency to develop cerebral infarction.

In a prospective study of Yamauchi et al. (19), the relation between the regional haemodynamic status of cerebral circulation and the subsequent risk of recurrent stroke in 40 patients with symptomatic internal carotid or middle cerebral arterial occlusive disease was evaluated. They all underwent PET and were divided into two groups: 33 patients with normal oxygen extraction fraction and 7 with misery perfusion. From the 33 patients only two suffered ipsilateral ischaemic stroke within the following year compared to 4 out of 7 with misery perfusion. The same author (18) published a case report of a patient with severe stenosis of the right intracranial internal carotid artery who presented with mild left hemiparesis resulting from a right frontal watershed infarct. PET 2 months after the stroke showed decreased cerebral blood flow with an increased oxygen extraction fraction in non infarcted areas of the affected hemisphere. Three months later he suffered a new infarct in the area exhibiting the highest oxygen extraction fraction.

These findings suggest that patients with major cerebral occlusive diseases and misery perfusion have a high risk for recurrent ischaemic stroke.

PET is the only tool to reliably and simultaneously measure metabolism and cerebral perfusion state. However, it is not generally available. Single Photon Emission Tomography (SPECT) also is a three dimensional imaging technique with reasonable accuracy. With tracers such as hexamethyl-propyl-eneamine oxime (HMPAO) or N-isopropyl-p-[^{123}I]-iodoamphetamine (^{123}-I-IMP), distribution of cerebral blood flow can be assessed. SPECT measurements performed at rest only yield little additional information in patients with carotid stenosis. However, also cerebral perfusion reserve can be assessed. Administration of acetazolamide or inhalation of carbon dioxide provokes an increase of blood flow via vasodilation. Patients with cerebral or carotid artery disease may show a blunted or absent response to acetazolamide (15). This occurs if the autoregulatory capacity is exhausted by reduced perfusion pressure distal to stenosis and poor collateral circulation. With the administration of acetazolamide the affected hemisphere or vascular distribution cannot further dilate while unaffected areas respond. This produces asymmetries in the distribution of the tracer, with increased retention in normally perfused areas.

Lord et al. (11) performed SPECT scanning with acetazolamide in 19 patients with carotid stenosis > 70 % before and after carotid reconstruction. They wanted to determine if the preoperative flow abnormalities were abolished by removing the obstruction. Nine patients demonstrated a perfusion defect ipsilateral to critical carotid stenosis. In 7 of them, SPECT study between 5 and 14 days after revascularisation showed improved or normal flow. The question whether acetazolamide reactivity on SPECT can also detect misery perfusion syndrome was addressed in two studies yielding conflicting results. Hirano et al. (8) found a significant correlation in a study of 14 patients between acetazolamide reactivity on ^{123}I-IMP SPECT and OEF and CBV/CBF as assessed with PET. Kuwabara et al. (9) did not find that correlation in HMPAO SPECT and PET in 7 patients.

Transcranial Doppler ultrasonography (TCD) is another powerful technology for noninvasive evaluation of cerebral haemodynamics. There is a good correlation between blood flow velocity measured by TCD and changes in cerebral blood flow measured by SPECT (4). Sugimori et al. designed a study (15) to determine whether TCD measurements correlate with PET measuremants of oxygen metabolism. In addition to flow velocity they also assessed cerebrovascular reserve by carbon dioxide inhalation during TCD measurement. Even though there was a good correlation between TCD and PET as far as blood flow is concerned, they failed to show a correlation between cerebrovascular reserve and oxygen metabolism or oxygen extraction fraction.

In conclusion, new developments in tomographic neuroimaging have made it possible to gain insight into the complex pathophysiological processes in cerebrovascular disease. There is sufficient evidence that there is a relationship between cerebral haemodynamic and metabolic status and symptoms and prognosis. As much knowledge as possible about the individual heamodynamic and metabolic profile as one component of a complex multifactorial disease could be helpful. Further studies need to be done in order to find out more about the contribution of those methods to clinical practice.

References

1. Baron JC, Bousser MG, Rey A, Guillard A, Comar D, Castaigne P (1981) Reversal of focal "Misery-Perfusion-Syndrome" by extra-intracranial arterial bypass in hemodynamic cerebral ischemia. Stroke 12: 454–459
2. Baron JC, Rougemont D, Bousser MG, Lebrun-Gandié P, Iba-Zizen MT, Chiras J (1983) Local CBF, oxygen extraction fraction (OEF), and $CMRO_2$: Prognostic value in recent supratentorial infarction in humans. J Cereb Blood Flow Metab 3 (Suppl 1): S1–S2
3. Burt RW, Witt RM, Cikrit DF, Reddy RV (1992) Carotid artery disease: Evaluation with acetazolamide-enhanced Tc-99m HMPAO SPECT. Radiology 182: 461–466
4. Dahl A, Russel D, Nyberg-Hansen R, Bakke SJ (1994) Cerebral vasoreactivity in unilateral carotid artery disease: a comparison of blood flow velocity and regional cerebral blood flow measurements. Stroke 25: 621–626
5. Duncan DB, Fink GR, Wirth M, Löttgen J, Pawlik G, Heiss WD (1996) Heterogeneity of hemodynamics and metabolism in patients with carotid artery disease. J Nucl Med 37: 429–432
6. Gibbs JM, Wise RJS, Leenders KL, Jones T (1984) Evaluation of cerebral perfusion reserve in patients with carotid-artery occlusion. Lancet I: 310–314
7. Heiss WD, Huber M, Fink GR, Herholz K, Pietrzyk U, Wagner R, Wienhard K (1992) Progressive derangement of periinfarct viable tissue in ischemic stroke. J Cereb Blood Flow Metab 12: 193–203
8. Hirano T, Minematsu K, Hasegawa Y, Tanaka Y, Hayashida K, Yamaguchi T (1994) Acetazolamide reactivity on 123-I-IMP Single Photon Emission Computed Tomography in patients with major cerebral artery occlusive disease: Correlation with Positron Emission Tomography parameters. J Cereb Blood Flow Metab 14: 763–770
9. Kuwabara Y, Ichiya Y, Sasaki M, Akashi Y, Yoshida T, Fukumura T, Masuda K, Fujii K, Fukui M (1994) Pre and postoperative evaluation of the perfusion reserve by acetazolamide 99mTc-HMPAO SPECT in patients with chronic occlusive cerebral arteries: a comparative study with PET. Kaku Igaku-Jen J Nuc Med 31: 1039–1050
10. Lassen NA (1966) The luxury-perfusion syndrome and its possible relation to acute metabolic acidosis localized within the brain. Lancet 2: 1113–1115
11. Lord RSA, Reid CVA, Ramsay SC, Yeates MG (1992) Unilateral carotid stenosis and impaired cerebral hemispheric vascular reserve. Ann Vasc Surg 6: 438–442
12. Powers WJ, Grubb RL Jr, Darriet D, Raichle ME (1985) Cerebral blood flow and cerebral metabolic rate of oxygen requirements for cerebral function and viability in humans. J Cereb Blood Flow Metab 5: 600–608
13. Powers WJ (1991) Cerebral hemodynamics in ischemic cerebrovascular disease. Ann Neurol 29: 231–240
14. Sacco RL, Ellenberg JH, Mohr JP, Tatemichi TK, Hier DB, Price TR, Wolf PA (1989) Infarcts of undetermined cause: the NINCDS stroke data bank. Ann Neurol 25: 382–390
15. Sugimori H, Ibayashi S, Fujii K, Sadoshima S, Kuwabara Y, Fujishima M (1995) Can transcranial doppler really detect reduced cerebral perfusion states. Stroke 26: 2053–2060
16. Vorstrup S (1988) Tomographic cerebral blood flow measurements in patients with ischemic cerebrovascular disease and evaluation of the vasodilatory capacity by the acetazolamide test. Acta Neurol Scand Suppl 114: 1–48

17. Wise RJS, Rhodes CG, Gibbs JM, Hatazawa J, Palmer T, Frackowiak RSJ, Jones T (1983) Disturbance of oxidative metabolism of glucose in recent human cerebral infarcts. Ann Neurol 14: 627–637
18. Yamauchi H, Fukuyama H, Fujimoto N, Nabatame H, Kimura J (1992) Significance of low perfusion with increased oxygen extraction fraction in a case of internal carotid artery stenosis. Stroke 23: 431–432
19. Yamauchi H, Fukuyama H, Nagahama Y, Nabatame H, Nakamura K, Yamamoto Y, Yonekura Y, Konishi J, Kimura J (1996) Evidence of misery perfusion and risk for recurrent stroke in major cerebral artery occlusive diseases from PET. J Neurol Neurosurg Psychiatry 61: 18–25

Author's address:
Dr. M. Grond
Max-Planck-Institut für Neurologische Forschung
Gleuelerstr. 50
50931 Köln, Germany

Regional anesthesia in carotid surgery: technique and results

A. M. Imparato, C. B. Rockman, T. S. Riles, M. Gold, P. J. Lamparello, G. Giangola, A. Ramirez, R. Landis

New York University Medical Center, New York, N.Y., USA

Introduction

It seems almost anachronistic at the end of the 20th century, which has enjoyed the most remarkable advances in general anesthetic techniques permitting the most daring, complex and time-consuming operations to be successfully performed in patients at high risk for developing devastating complications, to be presenting an operative experience during which local and regional anesthesia were preferentially used and considered to be superior to general anesthesia. The circumstances which led to this conclusion are in part the subject of this report as well as the currently employed technique for achieving the regional anesthesia required for the performance of deliberate, unhurried and precise reconstructions of the carotid and vertebral arteries in the neck.

Technique

The innervation of the neck which must be blocked with anesthetic agent to permit operations on the carotid arteries is primarily that emanating from nerve roots C2-C4. Additionally, the lower division of the trigeminal nerve may contribute to innervation of the lower border of the mandible thereby providing sensation at the upper end of a high neck incision, the lower neck may be innervated from T2, and the anterior neck may be partially innervated from the contralateral side. The carotid sheath contains sensory nerves via the ninth and tenth cranial nerves. Excellent anesthesia to permit carotid and even vertebral artery operations is obtained by blocking nerve roots C2-C4, supplementing the regional block with skin infiltration along the proposed line of incision as well as into the carotid sheath.

The anatomical landmarks which assist in locating the cervical nerve roots and the superficial cervical plexus which need to be blocked provide access primarily to the location of the nerve roots which enter the spinal canal by passing along the superior border of the cervical transverse processes. The notch of the thyroid cartilage marks the level of C4 while the cricoid marks the approximate level of the lower border of C6, also located from the point where the external jugular crosses the posterior border of the sternocleidomastoid muscle. Using these landmarks the lower border (C6) of the field and the upper border (C4) are marked. With the patients head turned to the contralateral side a line drawn from the cricoid cartilage to the point where the external jugular vein crosses the sternocleidomastoid muscle marks the level of C6 and a line parallel to this drawn from the notch of the thyroid cartilage delineates the level of C4. A point 1 cm posterior to the mastoid process is used to draw another line perpendicular to the C4 line. The point of crossing of these two lines at right angles marks the location of the transverse process of C4. C2 and C3 are located by marking the distance between the C4 and C6 lines previously drawn, cephalad along the line drawn from the C4 line to the mastoid process, thus establishing the level of the upper border of transverse process C2.

Having marked the locations of the transverse processes C2, 3, 4, 5cc of anesthetic agent is injected via a 22 gauge 1.5 inch needle at each of these three levels. The needle punctures are perpendicular to the skin. When bone is encountered the needle is "walked" off the bone cephalad penetrating beyond the bone no more than 1 to 2 mm. to thereby avoid either a subarachnoid or an intraarterial (vertebral artery) injection. Aspiration must be done and must prove to be dry before a slow injection is made, meanwhile communicating with the patient to detect changes in mental status which occur when either an intrathecal or an intraarterial injection has been made.

The superficial blocks are made along the anterior and posterior borders of the sternocleidomastoid muscle especially along its midlevels as well as along the lower border of the mandible.

Although a variety of anesthetic agents may be used for the cervical block 1.5 % mepivacaine with epinephrine 1:200,000 using 30 cc. total volume has provided anesthesia for almost 4 h with few problems, although because of the great vascularity of the neck systemic absorption and possible systemic toxicity must be anticipated in the rare patient. If anesthesia is to be supplemented during the procedure 1/2 % lidocaine with epinephrine is used for infiltration.

It is essential that the patients be sufficiently alert to respond to queries and that they be able to squeeze a sound producing toy placed in the hand corresponding to the carotid to the blocked. Sedation therefore is used sparingly. Additionally, the anticipated elevation of arterial blood pressure which often occurs on clamping the carotid, monitored through an intraarterial radial artery catheter placed in the contralateral wrist, must not be prevented from occuring for this often results in the appearance of cerebral ischemia in awake patients during the period when the carotid artery is clamped. On the few occasions when general anesthesia was needed in the middle of a procedure it has been induced together with tracheal intubation without difficulty.

Complications of cervical block

The untoward effects of cervical block anesthesia may come about as a result of systemic toxicity, from intrathecal injection, from injury to cranial nerves in the neck and from puncture of major vessels resulting in hematomas.

The central nervous system excitatory effects of local anesthetics may occur with or without intravascular injection of the agents, especially in an area as vascular as the neck where absorption may thereby be accelerated. There may occur seizures, tinnitus, sedation, manifestation of central nervous system effect or cardiac conduction blockade, arrhythmias, or even cardiac arrest, manifestations of effects on the cardiovascular system. It is therefore essential that individuals administering blocks be thoroughly familiar with the prevention and treatment of local anesthetic toxicity. Epinephrine used in conjunction with the anesthetic agents delays absorption and provides a measure of protection from systemic toxicity. The proximity of the vertebral arteries to the fields of injection means that there is the ever present hazard of intravascular injection, a hazard which can be minimized by limiting the penetration of the needles, by frequent aspirations during the advancement, by slow injections; maintaining close verbal contact with the patients to detect the earliest signs of toxicity, warning of the need to stop injecting.

Intrathecal injection results in a chain of signs beginning with progressive paralysis of the extremities, aphasia, loss of spontaneous responsiveness and unconsciousness, all in a period of minutes, requiring prompt intubation and ventilation until the effects of total spinal anesthesia dissipate, sometimes requiring hours.

Cranial nerve anesthetic blockade may result in transient hoarseness from which recovery usually occurs by the time the operation is completed, and rarely in transient tongue deviation from hypoglossal anesthesia especially if extensive local anesthetic supplemental infiltration is required during the procedure. Droop of the angle of the mouth may also occur transiently.

Method and results

The records of all patients undergoing carotid endarterectomy at the now New York University Medical Center between 1962 and 1994, 3975 in number, were retrospectively reviewed and analyzed with respect to demographics, indications for operations, anesthetic technique, be it general or local and outcome, which included neurologic complications whether transient or permanent, myocardial infarctions, whether clinically obvious or diagnosed by laboratory techniques and survival.

Local infiltration (1962 to 1970) or regional cervical block (1971 to 1994) was used in 3382 (85.1 %) operations in awake patients while 593 (14.9 %) operations were done under general anesthesia. The frequency of use of local or regional anesthesia was the same whether the indication for operation was preoperative transient ischemic attack (TIA), preoperative stroke or asymptomatic marked carotid stenosis or occlusion and ranged from 82.4 % to 88.4 %. There was, however, a higher incidence of contralateral carotid occlusions in the general anesthesia cohort (21.8 % vs. 15.4 %) compared to those done awake.

Analysis of anesthesia management during three time periods, 1962–1974 (no. 566), 1974–1984 (no. 1646), 1985–1994 (1763), shows a gradually increasing incidence of the use of general anesthesia, 10.6 %, 11.4 %, 19.8 %. This appears to have been a reflection of a greater use of routine or prophylactic shunting in patients with established neurologic deficits and in patients with contralateral occlusions. In 339 operations, 10 % of the awake series, intraarterial shunts were placed upon the appearance of signs of cerebral ischemia on test clamping, while in an additional 33 procedures shunts were placed electively for specific indications. Routine shunting was used with general anesthesia.

Transient and permanent cerebral neurologic complications totaled 2.2 % for the entire series with a trend towards fewer complications in the awake group compared to the general anesthesia group, (2.0 % vs. 3.2 %). A similar trend in favor of mortality occurred in the awake group, (1.4 %) against (2.0 %) for the general anesthesia group, although this did not achieve statistical significance. In the last period, 1975–1984, this difference in neurologic complications did, however, reach statistical significance, 1.2 % vs. 3.2 %, ($p < 0.01$).

Discussion

The decision to perform carotid artery endarterectomy in awake patients was made in 1962 when at the first workshop of the Joint Study of Extracranial Arterial Occlusion, the first prospective randomized clinical trial of the efficacy of carotid endarterectomy, it was apparent that the most experienced senior participants could not agree as to the hazards of carotid clamping, how best to monitor the reaction to clamping nor how to protect the brain against the anticipated clamping ischemia. As a junior participant with very limited experience, stimulated by the related experiences of Dr. E. Wiley, I decided to perform these operations under local anesthesia as a way of accurately monitoring the neurologic status of patients undergoing operations thus affording the opportunity to evaluate monitoring techniques as they became available, to test protective measures which were proposed and to accurately time and date the occurrence of any untoward events related to operations.

In rapid succession it was possible to demonstrate the unreliability of jugular venous oxygen levels, of early electroencephalography, and of carotid stump pressures as monitoring techniques while reenforcing the rapidity with which cerebral ischemic signs developed on carotid clamping, as rapidly as 10 s after application of occluding clamps with equally rapid recovery following their removal.

As protective measures the administration of carbonic anhydrase inhibitors or carbon dioxide inhalations to cause the cerebral vasodilatation associated with hypercarbia failed. Subsequently, induced hypocarbia was shown by Ehrenfeld to be equally ineffective. Only elevation of blood pressures sometimes to alarming levels and insertion of common carotid to internal carotid shunts rapidly deployed, reversed the ischemic signs which developed on carotid clamping in 7 % to 10 % of a mix of patients who came to operation for a variety of clinical and radiologic manifestations of cerebral ischemia. Artificial blood pressure elevation provoked myocardial ischemia and infarctions and so was used only to correct falling blood pressures. Inlying shunts sometimes created difficulties of exposure of the distal internal carotid arteries, were shown to be the pathways for emboli and sometimes became completely occluded and non functional from debris or thrombus in the common carotid artery (when direct puncture of the common artery was used for cerebral arteriography. Selective shunting minimized exposure and embolization problems, the entire routine permitting unhurried tension-free operations.

Test clamping the carotids in awake patients revealed that most patients who failed to tolerate clamping an isolated internal carotid artery (performed first), nevertheless tolerated clamping the isolated common carotid artery, remaining neurologically intact while the internal and external remained in communication. This led to a routine for shunt insertion in which the common carotid limb of the shunt is inserted first and rendered functional before reclamping the internal and external carotids for insertion of the upper limb of the shunt. On closure of the vessel after the endarterectomy advantage of these facts is taken to minimize ischemia.

Accurate assessment of the response to carotid clamping with subsequent review of the preoperative angiograms led to the appreciation of the concept of carotid predominance and the importance of visualization of the posterior communicating artery in predicting whether carotid clamping will be tolerated.

Perhaps the greatest lesson learned was that the causes of perioperative neurologic events could be accurately diagnosed in 80 % of instances when they occured, that technical factors predominated, sharing equal incidences with other causes. Operative site thrombosis, intraoperative embolization, intracerebral hemorrhage and clamping ischemia occurred with equal frequencies and each of these frequencies was equal to a fifth group in which precise diagnosis was not possible. It is felt that this alone, which emphasizes the great importance of attention to the technical details of the performance of the operation, has contributed more to improving the safety of the operations than any other factor.

Insofar as the conclusions to be drawn from the analysis of three decades of operative experience with carotid endarterectomy, one can only be impressed with the facts that no steep learning curve has been involved in achieving the rather consistent results. Seven vascular surgeons trained in the basics of performing the operation in awake patients following a relatively uniform routine have contributed to the series starting from their first days as attending surgeons on the Vascular Service at the New York University Hospital (now Tisch Hospital of the New York University Medical Center). The differences in event rates between regional and general anesthesia are too small to accurately assess in a retrospective review of a more than a three-decade experience. The differences, however, may be of major importance in a surgical endeavor in which operative complications have the potential of being reduced to an irreducible minimum, perhaps to less than 1 % in the mixed population requiring operation. Only a prospective randomized clinical trial would have the statistical power to resolve the issue in spite of the fact that a number of other anesthetic routines are reported to yield excellent results.

In terms of series which compare the results of regional and general anesthesia as variables in the performance of CAE. There is no agreement as to whether in non-randomized trials stroke rates, myocardial infarctions or survival are significantly different between the two approaches. There appear to be as many favoring regional anesthesia as reporting no differences. Our own experience, however, indicates that the incidence of stroke attributable to clamping ischemia is about 0.5 % and should be almost entirely preventable. Whether strokes which might occur under general anesthesia are due to interference by a shunt, because of embolization through a shunt, because of unease on the part of a surgeon not knowing the condition of a patient presenting with a technically difficult and time-consuming operation can only be determined by a thorough analysis of the circumstances and findings related to the events.

Although only of documentary value, a number of surgeons who having begun their experience with carotid endarterectomy in generally anesthetized patients have then changed to operating in awake patients have reported that they operate with greater confidence at a more deliberate pace knowing the precise condition of the patient. They also report rather marked differences in the postoperative appearances of operated patients in favor of those having been operated awake.

Conclusions

Regional anesthesia offers the vascular surgeon a modality which allows the achievement of excellent clinical results while permitting unhurried and precise operations on the carotid arteries when combined with selective shunting. It permits the most accurate direct monitoring of the neurologic status of patients undergoing operation, so that selective corrective measures can be instituted upon the appearance of neurologic abnormalities. Accurate timing of the occurrence of events, specifically thereby making possible the differential diagnosis between intraoperative embolization and clamping ischemia, combined with other diagnostic measures, provides an accurate performance profile for each surgeon who can then make appropriate adjustments in technique. Whether regional anesthesia is clearly superior to general anesthesia in neurologic and cardiac morbidity and mortality should be the subject of a prospective randomized trial.

References

1. Spencer FC, Eisemann B (1962) Technique of carotid endarterectomy. Surg Gynecol Obstet 115: 115–117
2. Imparato AM, Ramirez A, Riles TS, Mintzer R (1982) Cerebral protection in carotid surgery. Arch Surg 117: 1073
3. Riles TS, Gold M (1997) Alternatives to general anesthesia for carotid endarterectomy. In: Moore WS (ed) Surgery for Cerebrovascular Disease. 2nd edition. Philadelphia: WB Saunders, Co., in press
4. Riles TS, Imparato AM, Jacobowitz GR et al. (1994) The cause of perioperative stroke after carotid endarterectomy. J Vasc Surg 19: 206–216
5. Imparato AM (1993) Cerebral protection during anesthesia for carotid and vertebral surgery. In: Bernstein EF, Callow AD, Nicolaides AN et al. (eds) Cerebral Revascularisation. London: Med-Orion Publishing Company, p 405
6. Imparato AM (1996) Carotid endarterectomy: Indications and techniques for carotid surgery. In: Haimovici H, Ascer E, Hollier LH et al. (eds) Haimovici's Vascular Surgery, Fourth Edition. Boston: Blackwell Science, Inc.
7. Imparato AM (1988) Extracranial vascular disease: advances in operative indications and techniques. World J Surg 12: 756
8. Imparato AM, Riles TS, Ramirez AA, Lamparello PJ, Mintzer R (1985) Anaesthetic management in carotid artery surgery. Aust NZ J Surg 55: 315–319
9. Connolly JE (1985) Carotid endarterectomy in the awake patient. Am J Surg 150: 159–165
10. Donato AT, Hill SL (1992) Carotid arterial surgery using local anesthesia: a private practice retrospective study. Am Surg 446–450
11. Hafner CD, Evans WE (1988) Carotid endarterectomy with local anesthesia: results and advantages. J Vasc Surg 7: 232–239
12. Rich NM, Hobson RW II (1975) Carotid endarterectomy under regional anesthesia. Am Surg 253–258
13. Benjamin ME, Silva MB, Watt C (1993) Awake patient monitoring to determine the need for shunting during carotid endarterectomy. Surgery 114: 673–681
14. Allen BT, Anderson CB, Rubin BG et al. (1994) The influence of anesthetic technique on perioperative complications after carotid endarterectomy. J Vasc Surg 19: 834–843
15. Muskett A, McGreevy J, Miller M (1986) Detailed comparison of regional and general anesthesia for carotid endarterectomy. Am J Surg 152: 691–694
16. Gabelman CG, Gann DS, Ashworth CJ (1983) One hundred consecutive carotid reconstructions: local versus general anesthesia. Am J Surg 145: 477–482
17. Corson JD, Chang BB, Shah DM (1987) The influence of anesthetic choice on carotid endarterectomy outcome. Arch Surg 122: 807–812
18. Peitzman AB, Webster MW, Loubeau JM (1982) Carotid endarterectomy under regional (conductive) anesthesia. Ann Surg 196: 59–64
19. Andersen CA, Rich NM, Collins GJ, McDonald PT (1980) Carotid endarterectomy: regional versus general anesthesia. Ann Surg 46: 323–327
20. Bergeron P, Benichou H, Rudondy P, Jausseran JM, Ferdani M, Courbier R (1991) Stroke prevention during carotid surgery in high risk patients (value of transcranial Doppler and local anesthesia). J Cardiovasc Surg 32: 713–719
21. Becquemin JP, Paris E, Valverde A, Pluskwa F, Melliere D (1991) Carotid surgery. Is regional anesthesia always appropriate? J Cardiovasc Surg 32: 592–598
22. Shah DM, Darling RC III, Chang BB, Bock DEM, Paty PSK, Leather RP (1994) Carotid endarterectomy in awake patients: its safety, acceptability, and outcome. J Vasc Surg 19: 1015–1020
23. Callow AD, Matsumoto G, Baker D et al. (1978) Protection of the high risk carotid endarterectomy patients by continuous electroencephalography. J Cardiovasc Surg 19: 55
24. Hertzer NR, Avellone JC, Farrell CJ (1984) The risk of vascular surgery in a metropolitan community. J Vasc Surg 1: 13–21
25. Fode NC, Sundt TM Jr, Robertson JT, Peerless SJ, Shields CB (1986) Multicenter retrospective review of results and complications of carotid endarterectomy in 1981. Stroke 17: 370–374

26. Moore WS, Yee JM, Hall AD (1973) Collateral cerebral blood pressure: An index of tolerance to temporary carotid occlusion. Arch Surg 106: 520
27. Towne JB, Bernhard WM (1982) Neurologic deficit following carotid endarterectomy. Surg Gynecol Obstet 154: 849
28. Imparato AM (1989) Is there a need for prospective randomized clinical trials of carotid endarterectomy. In: Veith FJ (ed) Current critical problems in vascular surgery. St. Louis: Quality Medical Publishing, p 553

Author's address:
A. M. Imparato, M.D.
New York University Medical Center
530 First Avenue, Suite 6F
New York, N.Y. 10016, USA

Perioperative results of carotid endarterectomy with cervical epidural anesthesia

B. Habozit, J. P. Derosier, A. Gaillard

Head of Department of Vascular Surgery

Much has been written on the monitoring and protection of the brain during surgery of the carotid bifurcation. Controversy exists about whether to use an intraluminal shunt during carotid cross-clamping. In this controversy surgeons adhere to one of three policies: routine shunting, no shunting at all, and selective shunt. Cerebral ischemia secondary to cross-clamping of the carotid bifurcation is one of the causes of operative strokes. Behaviour of the awake patient is a safe and practical method; it permits selective shunting with good specificity and sensitivity in detecting neurological events. For all these reasons, we chose cervical epidural anesthesia (CEA) which was described in the English literature as early as 1933 by Dogliotti (4) and used for carotid surgery in 1963 by Green (6). We introduced CEA for carotid endarterectomy in France in 1984 (7). CEA offers a combination of profound anesthesia and muscular relaxation of the cervical region. The method is not difficult and can be performed by any anesthetist skilled in epidural anesthesia of the lumbar region; by attention to the details of epidural anesthesia technique, complications can be avoided. The effectiveness of analgesia was usually excellent, and operating on a awake patient is not a burden to either the surgeon or the patient. In order to evaluate perioperative complications, 628 carotid endarterectomies were included in a retrospective study, between January 1984 and January 1996.

Technique of cervical epidural anesthesia and postoperative care

The cervical plexus is formed by the ventral primary rami of the first four cervical nerves. Each nerve divides into an ascending and descending branch which communicates with the nerves above and below respectively; these series of nerve loops form the cervical plexus. The first cervical nerve has no cutaneous distribution, although the others do. The major cutaneous branches of interest are the lesser occipital nerve, the greater auricular nerve, and the supraclavicular nerve. Of the muscular branches the most important is the phrenic nerve. Other motor branches supply the muscles of the neck including the scalenes.

For the induction of anesthesia the patient is lightly premedicated (alprazolam) and has been prepared by a discussion prior to operation. Upon entering the anesthesic area, appropriate intravenous line is established to provide access for fluids and drugs; colloid infusion was started off before the epidural puncture; the usual monitoring for carotid surgery included electrocardiogram (lead CM5), automatic control of arterial blood pressure and digital oxymetry. The patient is positioned in a sitting position with the back quite straight and the neck acutely flexed. The most easily palpable interspace at the base of the neck is chosen; it is usually between the sixth and the seventh cervical vertebrae or the seventh cervical and the first thoracic. The technique of accomplishing the puncture should be that with which the anesthetist is most familiar. After cutaneous local anesthesia, an 18-gauge Tuohy needle is advanced by a midline approach into the chosen epidural space, the bevel being pointed in a cephalad direction; the tip of the needle enters the epidural space obliquely and an move further into the space before impinging upon the dura; careful aspiration ensures that the needle had not entered the subarachnoid space nor penetrated an epidural vein. The ligaments of the cervical region are softer than those of the lumbar region; for this reason it is recommended that a hanging drop technique or similar technique of presence of negative pressure be the method of choice for identification of cervical epidural space. From then, a catheter is introduced through the needle, directed cephalad, and passed for about 8 cms beyond the tip of the needle. After withdrawal of the needle, the catheter is secured in the usual manner. The patient is returned in supine position and a test dose of 3 ml of 3 % bupivacaîne is injected through the catheter. In the absence of signs of systemic vascular absorption or inadvertent intrathecal injection, the definitive dose of local anesthesic is injected: 12 to 15 ml of 0.4 per cent bupivacaine with 5 gammas per ml of fentanyl. The patient is then placed during 15 min in declive position with rotation in the side of surgical procedure. Surgical procedure may begin 30 min after injection of local anaesthesic. Patients are carefully observed for loss of consciousness, somnolence and neurological deficit of the hand and the arm, during all the operation and in the recovery room. Blood pressure and heart rate are monitored during the first 24 h postoperatively. Electrocardiogram and myocardial enzymes are obtained during the three first postoperative days and at the end of the hospital stay.

Technique of carotid endarterectomy

"Gentle" is the key word for dissecting the carotid bifurcation. After proximal control of the common carotid artery (CCA) is obtained, distal control of the internal carotid artery (ICA) is likewise obtained away from the carotid bifurcation; after distal control, careful palpation of the distal artery is carried out to assure the surgeon he is distal to any unsuspected tongue of atheroma; this will permit him to clamp away from the end point of the endarterectomy. Finally, the external carotid artery (ECA) is dissected with the superior thyroid artery, without dissection of the tissue directly at the crotch between ICA and ECA; the surrounding structures (internal jugular and nerves) are dissected away from the ICA, leaving the carotid bulb undisturbed. The patient is systematically given 5000 to 8000 units of heparin and the common, internal and external carotid arteries were clamped. Dissection of the bulb is completed after cross-clamping. Standard endarterectomy of the ICA requires usually 2.5X magnification loops. The plane between the atheroma and the artery is usually easily found and circumferential dissection is performed; the surgeon should attempt to render the same technical precision to the ECA as he does in performing the ICA; the distal end point of the atheroma in the ICA is the crucial part of the operation: done properly, the intima will separate sharply and a perfect end point will be obtained so that distal "tacking sutures" are unnecessary. Prior to closure, the endarterectomy site was irrigated with heparinized saline and smaller debris were identified by rubbing the surface with fine, wet gauze. This study comprised 509 standard endarterectomies with longitudinal arteriotomy extending the last 3 cm of the CCA to the ICA beyond the termination of the plaque. Simple closure with 7–0 monofilament suture was done in 480 cases and with Dacron-patch in 29. Eversion endarterectomy was the routine technique in patients with elongation of the ICA since 1984 (46 cases); in patients with a plaque that does not extend high in the ICA, eversion endarterectomy was done through the CCA since 1991 (55 cases). In 18 patients, fragility of arteries after endarterectomy or neck fibrosis prescribed to realize a bypass technique, with saphenous vein (??) or thin-walled PTFE (7). Technical perfection continues to be the factor of greatest importance in the avoidance of stroke during carotid endarterectomy. Because most complications from endarterectomy are of technical nature, it makes sense to ensure the correctness of the procedure after its completion. I have no experience with intraoperative arteriogram and little with angioscopy (112 cases).

The use of a temporary indwelling shunt enables interruption of ipsilateral cerebral hemisphere flow for only the time it takes to insert and extricate the shunt, usually 2 to 3 min. I use Javid shunt, with a bulbous enlargement at each end that discourages dislodgement when special clamps are applied; technical perfection rather than speed is to be emphasized to insert the shunt into the ICA. In my practice, the selective use of the shunt was based upon the occurrence of neurological events during carotid cross-clamping. Usually, a temporary clamping of 1 min is used in order to detect if the patient is in need of a shunt. However, in our study, it was shown that the 1-min clamping did not reveal all those patients in need of an intraoperative shunt and there were patients who still experienced a functional ischemia after more than 10 min.

The indication for carotid endarterectomy was hemispheric transcient ischemic attack (including amaurosis fugax) in 324, vertebrobasilar transcient ischemic attack in 69, hemispheric stroke a variable amount of recovery in 97; 138 patients were asymptomatic. Bilateral operations (142) were staged within a week in 91 cases, or during the run-off in 51; patients with staged bilateral procedures have been recorded twice, since they have been exposed twice to risk. A fairly high percentage of the patients showed signs of coronary disease (42 % of patients).

Perioperative results

Nine-hundred-forty-two consecutive carotid endarterectomies were performed between January 1984 and January 1994. These operations were performed by the same vascular team composed of one vascular surgeon (BH) and two anesthetists. CEA was performed for 628 operations on 486 patients. The mean age was 69.9 years, with a range of 33 to 88 years. Selective shunt was inserted in 52 patients (8.3 %). The average operation time was 41 min, with an average cross-clamping time of 14. Of the 628 carotid endarterectomies, 625 resulted in no peri-operative deficit and three developed a minor temporary neurologic deficit (0.5 %). No perioperative myocardial infarction was observed.

The effectiveness of CEA was excellent, without additional analgesia, during 578 surgical procedures (92 %); 50 patients received small doses of IV benzodiazepines or narcotics with additional in situ local 2 % lidocaine, but verbal communication was always maintained. No patient required additional epidural injection and no general anesthesia was required. If the identification of the epidural space was successful in all the patients of the study, epidural puncture was unsuccessful (arthrosis) in 16 patients during the same 12-year period. Epidural venipuncture occurred in 17 cases (2.7 %), prescribing a second puncture in the adjacent spinal interspace. One of the first patients of the study developed progressive respiratory failure with anesthesia of the phrenic nerves: the solution consisted of 0.5 per cent lidocaine and has been modified in the remainder. CEA was used without complication in 61 patients with severe chronic obstructive pulmonary disease. Systolic arterial pressure decreased by more than 30 % of the preanesthesic value in 59 operations (9.4 %) and was treated with IV ephedrine; decreases in heart rate to less than 45 were present in 22 procedures (3.5 %) and were pomptly treated with IV atropine. Severe hypertension during carotid cross-clamping was observed in 57 procedures (9 %) and was corrected with IV clonidine, labetalol or trinitrine; moderate hypertension was observed in 201 procedures, without treatment. No myocardial infarction occurred during CEA; patients with coronary disease received systematically IV trinitrine during operation.

For neurological outcome, neurological events were separated into two categories: immediate perioperative deficits and delayed deficits; delayed deficits were due to postoperative events (thrombosis, hyperperfusion...) and cannot be blamed on operative ischemia. Before carotid clamping, a transcient decreased level of consciousness occurred in two patients (0.3 %); in addition, transient hemispheric attack was noticed within 1 min of carotid declamping in one patient. During carotid clamping, 94 neurological events occurred (15 %), whether immediately after cross-clamping (50) or later (44), from 5 to 15 min after the beginning of cross-clamping. The use of temporary indwelling shunt was effective in all the patients (50) with early deficit and in 2 patients with late deficit: a minor deficit persisted after operation in 3 patients (0.5 %); in other cases, neurological status was perfect after restoration of flow (either shunting or declamping). No perioperative acute stroke occurred during 628 procedures. In fact, CEA permitted a selective shunting in 52 carotid endarterectomies of the 628 operations, i.e. 8.3 % of all the procedures.

Postoperatively until the 30th day, four patients (0.8 % of patients) died of stroke with large ischemic (two patients) or hemorrhagic (two patients) strokes: the surgical procedures have been uneventful and did not require a shunt in every case. Three patients suffered established strokes of minor degree (0.6 % of patients), with normal carotid in one case and with thrombus in two (two removed). One patient died of sudden asystole 6 days after the procedure, probably a coronary death (0.2 %); a myocardial infarction occurred in one patient 3 days after surgery (0.2 % of patients).

Discussion

Local or regional anesthesia has been used for carotid endarterectomy since the beginning of carotid surgery (8). CEA is a regional anesthesia used by our team since 1984; during the first 3 years of this study, selection for CEA was used only in elderly patients and in high-risk patients with signs and/or cerebral sequelae visible on CT-scan and those with controlateral occlusive disease and/or non-functional cerebral arteries; good practice and results induced us to propose CEA for every patient since 1987. The results of this study indicate that prevention of perioperative stroke during carotid endarterectomy is feasible; the major causes of stroke are poor surgical technique and lowered intracerebral flow after carotid clamping; postoperative strokes were intimal flaps in only two patients (0.4 % of patients).

The technique of CEA appears to be simple and successful in the majority of the patients. The handing-drop technique, performed in the sitting position, allowed ready identification of the cerival epidural space. Diffusion of the local anesthetic solution in the cephalad direction within the skull is precluded by the adhesion of the meningeal dura to the endosteal dura. The thickness of the dura mater which is 2.5 mm at the cervical level versus 0.5 mm at lumbar may account for the infrequency of dural puncture; the venipuncture may occur, easily documented by aspiration through the Tuohy needle. We did not observe epidural hematoma when heparin is given before carotid clamping, about 45 min after epidural puncture. Two larger series of 3164 and 950 anticoagulated patients selected for vascular surgery with epidural or spinal anesthesia were reported to be free of such complication (9, 11).

The phrenic nerve conduction and the intercostal muscle function may be exceptionaly impaired by CEA (lidocaine); fentanyl combined with bupivacaine rather depressed ventilation (14). CEA induces cardiac sympathetic blockade with decrease of arterial blood pressure and heart rate (1) as the incidence of myocardial ischemia (12). A decrease in blood pressure may compromise cerebral and coronary perfusion and have to be corrected; conversely, moderate hypertension is unusual and does not prevent cerebral ischemia during carotid clamping in patients with critically impaired collateral function; severe hypertension is always corrected with IV drugs; perioperative hypertension in carotid surgery is usually best correlated with badly controlled preoperative hypertension. Usual stability of the systemic blood pressure is observed with CEA, especially after carotid declamping (3). We observed a 0.4 % incidence of postoperative myocardial infarction which is less than the 10 – 18.2 % incidence reported in high-risk patients operated upon under general anesthesia (5).

For CEA, the patient is neurologically monitored during the clamping of the carotid bifurcation; a shunt is used in cases of neurological dysfunction. Local anesthesia has been used since the 1960s and Spencer and Eiseman (13) blowed the safety of selective shunting. Now, most surgeons are said to opt for general anesthesia, but carotid surgery under regional anesthesia has some advantages for patients at risk of tolerance to cross-clamping (clinical signs and/or cerebral sequelae) and patients with coronary artery disease. The 15.5 % of neurological deficits observed in this study during carotid endarterectomy with CEA is significantly lower than suspected cases of ischemia detected in patients being operated on under general anesthesia; a great number of methods has been used for neurological monitoring in these patients: stump pressure, rCBF measurements, EEG, transcranial Doppler alone or together with evoked potential response, jugular vein O_2 tension, and subjectively estimated quality of the back bleeding from the stump; transcranial Doppler seems to be the most versatile and practible of available methods. There is a small group, 5 – 10 % of the patients, who needs the shunt. In fact, shunt is obviously unnecessary in most patients and shunt may not function properly or may be responsible for embolization or intimal injury; finally, shunt may increase the difficulty of the operation. It has been shown that patients with controlateral carotid occlusion and those with a preoperative stroke are in need of a shunt more often than other patients (8); analysis of preoperative anatomic lesions of carotid arteries in our study showed that shunt was used in 6 % of procedures in patients with unilateral lesion, 12 % with controlateral stenosis and 19 % with contralateral occlusion.

Comparative study with cervical block shows that there is not an important difference with CEA; the purpose is the same: selective shunting (2, 10). CEA allows reoperation for postoperative thrombosis or controlateral carotid endarterectomy within 1 week, if epidural catheter has been secured after operation. CEA is a simple technique, easy to perform by trained anesthetists with low incidence of complications or side-effects such as hypotension and bradycardia; this technique should be considered as an alternative to cervical block for carotid artery surgery.

References

1. Bonnet F, Szekely B, Abhay K et al. (1989) Baroreceptors control after cervical epidural anesthesia in patients undergoing carotid artery surgery. J Cardiovasc Anesth 3: 418–24
2. Connolly J (1985) Carotid endarterectomy in the awake patient. Am J Surg 150: 159–65
3. Corson J, Chang B, Leopold P et al. (1986) Perioperative hypertension in patients undergoing carotid endarterectomy: shorter duration under regional block anesthesia. Circulation (suppl I): I.1–I.4
4. Dogliotti AM (1993) Segmental peridural anesthesia. Am J Surg 20: 107–9
5. Ennix CL Jr, Lawrie GM, Morris GC et al. (1981) Improved results of carotid endarterectomy in patients with symptomatic coronary disease; an analysis of 1546 consecutive carotid operations; Stroke 10: 122–5
6. Green CD (1962) Cervical epidural anesthesia for carotid endarterectomy. Surg Gynecol Obstet 117: 366–7
7. Habozit B, Derosier JP, Gaillard A (1985) Anesthésie péridurale cervicale et chirurgie carotidienne et ver-tébrale. Lyon Chir 1: 64–7
8. Imparato AM, Ramirez A, Riles T, Mintzer R (1982) Cerebral protection in carotid surgery. Arch Surg 117: 1073–8
9. Odoon JA, Sih IL (1983) Epidural analgesia and anticoagulant therapy. Experience with one thousand cases of continuous epidural. Anaesthesia 38: 254–9
10. Peitzman AB, Webster MW, Loubeau JM et al. (1982) Carotid endarterectomy under regional (conduc-tive) anesthesia. Ann Surg 196: 59–94
11. Rao TKL, El-Etr AA (1981) Anticoagulation following placement of epidural and subarachnoid catheters. Anesthesiology 55: 618–20
12. Reiz S, Balfors E (1982) Coronary hemodynamic effects of general anesthesia and surgery. Reg Anesth 7 (suppl): S8–S18
13. Spencer F, Eiseman B (1962) Technique of carotid endarterectomy. Surg Gynecol Obstet 115: 115–7
14. Takasaki M, Takahashi T (1980) Respiratory function during cervical and thoracic extradural analgesia in patients with normal lungs. Br J Anesth 52: 1271–5

Author's address:
B. Habozit, MD
Head of Department
of Vascular Surgery
Boulevard Massenet 306
73000 Chambéry, France

Local anesthesia and intraoperative quality control in carotid surgery

G. W. Hagmüller, G. Hastermann, H. Ptakovsky

1. Chirurgische Abteilung Wilhelminenspital der Stadt Wien, Wien, Austria
(Head: Univ.-Prof. Dr. Georg W. Hagmüller)

Since indication for carotid endarterectomy in symptomatic as well as in asymptomatic patients is well defined by recent randomised clinical studies (NASCET, ECST, ACAS) our aim must be to reduce perioperative mortality and morbidity to acceptable limits. To show significant benefits of surgical therapy during the first 2 years, it is necessary to reach a stroke rate/death rate of less than 3 %.

By means of intraoperative quality control with SEP's, stump pressure measurement or EEG controls in operations performed in general anesthesia or neuromonitoring during operations performed in loco-regional anesthesia combined complication rates less than 3 % can be reached.

This report details the technique of carotid endarterectomy in loco-regional anesthesia which appears to reach those acceptable limits of risk in a consecutive series of 382 patients and discusses the results.

Materials and methods

Between October 1, 1992 and June 30, 1995 the authors performed 382 carotid endarterectomies with a total of 475 supraaortic extra thoracic arterial reconstructions using cervical block and local anesthesia, neuromonitoring on the awake patients and selective shunting exclusively with straight Argyl-shunts. All patients were informed of the procedure, no conversion to general anesthesia was necessary.

Technique:

After premedication with 7.5 mg Midazolam (Dormicum), a superficial and deep cervical blockade at C3, C4 and C5 level with 30 cc 1 % Lidocain as a maximum is performed by the surgeon or anesthesiologist. Unilateral surgical exposure for carotid endarterectomy or even transposition of the subclavian or vertebral artery can be performed by this kind of anesthesia. Perioperative neuromonitoring includes constant registration of the consciousness of the patient and motion of the contralateral hand by a squeezable puppet. Continuous arterial blood pressure- and ECG-monitoring is mandatory.

Following data were prospectively documented in all patients on a specific patient protocol:
1. Side of cerebral symptoms

2. Side of operation

3. Angiomorphology (ACI-stenosis 0 – 100 %)
   a) of the operated ACI
   b) of the contralateral ACI

4. Perioperative cerebral reaction during clamping
   a) no reaction   c) complete unconsciousness
   b) slight unconsciousness   d) contralateral paresis ("stop squeezing")

5. Use of an indwelling shunt (yes / no)

6. Blood pressure reaction
   a) during clamping
   b) during whole operation

7. Operating surgeon

8. Operative technique
   a) Eversionendarterectomy (EEA)
   b) Conventional endarterectomy (TEA)
      aa) with patch (saphenous- / external jugular "sleeve patch" / PTFE-patch)
      bb) direct suture
   c) miscellaneous

Results

382 operations were performed by eight surgeons (five seniors, three residents) with an individual distribution: 142 – 82 – 45 – 31 – 30 – 30 – 22 and 5 operations. During 58 operations (15 %) immediate shunting within the first minute of clamping because of positive neuromonitoring was necessary. By means of this immediate shunting complete cerebral recovery occurred in 44 patients, prolonged cerebral recovery in nine patients (2.35 %). Five patients suffered a lethal perioperative cerebral complication, four infarctions and one intracerebral hemorrhage. Postoperatively two more patients died of myocardial infarction.

The overall mortality was 1.8 % (seven patients), stroke related mortality 1.3 % (five patients). The combined complication rate (stroke / mortality) was 4.2 % for 382 carotid endarterectomies in 126 asymptomatic and 256 symptomatic patients with an ACI-stenosis exceeding 60 %. There was no significant difference of complications between the asymptomatic and symptomatic group in this rather small series.

In this prospective study an evaluation between different techniques of endarterectomies could be studied: Eversionendarterectomy versus conventional endarterectomy with patch plasty of the ACI.

Two-hundred-three EEA and 162 conventional TEA were performed. Twenty-seven miscellaneous operations as recurrent stenosis resection with graft interposition or TEAs with direct suture complete the 382 operations (Fig. 1).

Because of individual surgical experience and sometimes local morphological convenience a randomization for these two techniques of carotid endarterectomy could not be performed.

The mortality in both groups was equal with 1.9 %, the stroke rate in the "patch group" with 3.3 %, versus 1.9 % in the EEA-group nearly double as high but not statistically different (Student t-test p-0.02 (Fig. 2).

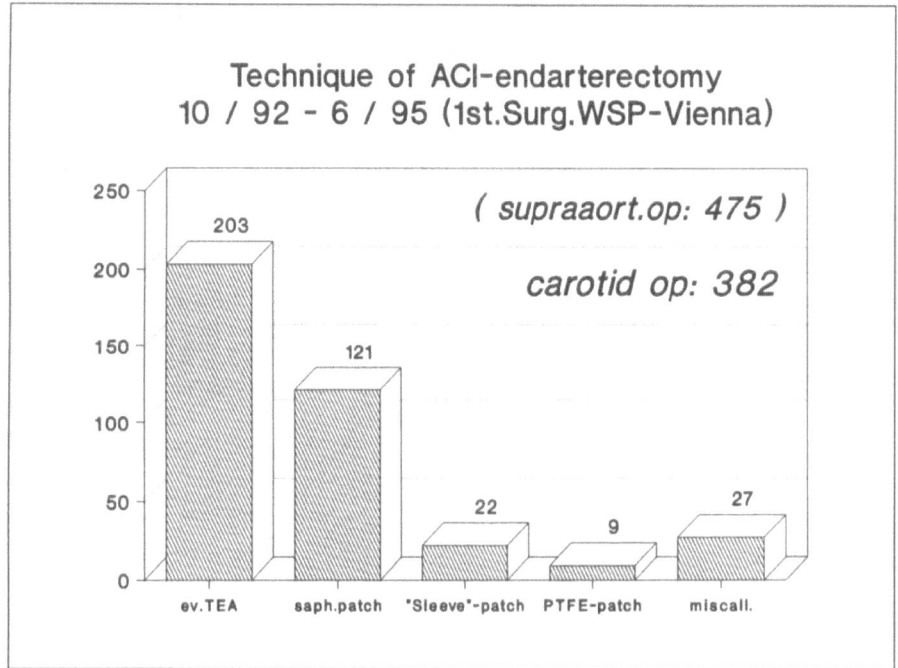

Fig. 1

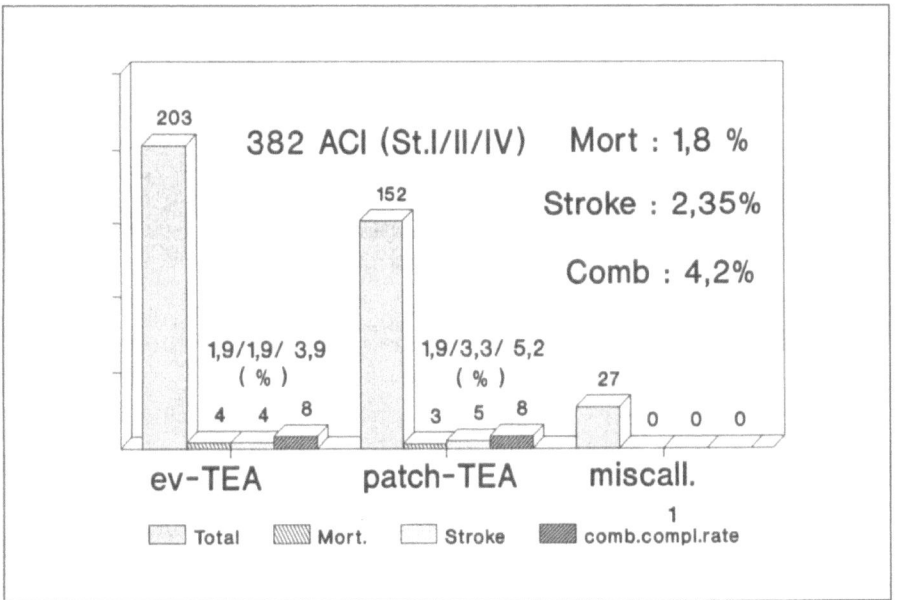

Fig. 2

External Jugular vein "Sleeve patch":

Because of inconvenience, harvesting a saphenous vein patch at the ankle or groin region in local anesthesia and of, sometimes, wound healing complications at these harvesting areas a new technique of vein patching was developed.

An adequate length of the external jugular vein can be saved subcutaneously from the neck incision for carotid artery exposure. The external jugular is not tailored like a usual vein patch by longitudinal incision, but is turned inside out like a sleeve. By this you get a tubed "double vein patch" which is endothelized all around.

Care must be taken during suturing the proximal and distal ends of the "sleeve patch" into the edges of the arteriotomy to be sure both blades of the patch are stitched thoroughly through. In this series 22 "sleeve patches" could be inserted with no early or late complication such as suture line bleeding or aneurysmal patch degeneration. All patients were controlled by duplex scanning 3, 6 and 12 months postoperatively.

Discussion

Published date of the last 5 years (NASCET, ECST, V.A.-study, ACAS-study) recommend carotid endarterectomy for the prevention of stroke in patients who have a 60 % or greater stenosis, symptomatic or asymptomatic, documented by angiography, if there are no serious medical problems to contraindicate the procedure. In the ACAS-study it is stated that the benefits derived from the operation are dependent upon surgeons having documented a perioperative mobidity and mortality of less than 3 %.

Recommended acceptable limits of combined morbidity and mortality due to stroke during a following endarterectomy are listed in Table 1. The aim must be to reach a near zero complication rate by not excluding high-risk patients from the benefit of this operation. In our series of 382 carotid endarterectomies for stroke prevention no patient was excluded because of "high risk" (age, myocardial, pulmonal, cerebral, cancer).

By means of regional anesthesia the perioperative medical risk could be reduced to 1.04 % myocardial infarctions, two of them ended lethally (0.52 %) and the lethal cerebral risk to 1.3 %. So the total mortality was 1.8 %. Nine patients (2.35 %) suffered a perioperative stroke with good recovery tendency and no disabling sequalea. All but one of these nine patients had a positive preoperative CCT.

The most sensitive parameter of cerebral dysfunction due to oxygen reduction caused by clamping the carotid artery is the evaluation of consciousness by perioperative

Table 1. Recommended acceptable limits of combined morbidity and mortality due to stroke during ACI-endarterectomy

▶ Asymptomatic stenosis	3 %
▶ Transient ischemic attacks	5 %
▶ Previous ischemic stroke	7 %
▶ Recurrent ischemic stenosis	10 %
▶ Mortality for all groups	2 %

(From NASCET 1991, JAMA 1995. Am J Med 1988)

neuromonitoring. This seems to be easier to handle and superior to registered SEPs or EEG-monitoring to select patients who need a shunt. Operating on an awake patient sharpens the mind of the surgical team for immediate reaction if the patient shows discomfort or clinical signs of stroke. Furthermore, the ongoing attempt for atraumatic operative technique which reduces "per se" perioperative complication rate is inspired.

References

1. Anthony T, Johansen K (1994) Optimal outcome for "high-risk" carotid endarterectomy. Am J Surg 167: 469–71
2. Bergeron P, Benichou H, Rudondy P et al. (1991) Stroke prevention during carotid surgery in high risk patients. J cardiovasc Surg 32: 713–9
3. Davies MJ, Murell GC, Cronin KD et al. (1990) Carotid endarterectomy under cervical plexus block: a prospective clinical audit, Anaest Intensive Care 18: 219–23
4. European Carotid Surgery Trialists Collaborative Group (1991) MRC European Carotid Surgery Trial. Interim results for symptomatic patients with severe (70 – 99 %) or with mild (0 – 29 %) carotid stenosis. Lancet 337: 1235–43
5. Executive Committee for the Asymptomatic Carotid Atherosclerosis Study. Endarterectomy for asymptomatic carotid artery stenosis. JAMA 273: 1421–8
6. Fried KS, Elias SM, Raggi R (1990) Carotid endarterectomy under locak anesthesia. N Eng J Med 87: 795–7
7. North American Symptomatik Carotid Endarterectomy Trial Collaborators. Beneficial effect of carotid endarterectomy in symtomatic patients with high-grade carotid stenosis. New Engl J Med 325: 445–507
8. Pruitt JC (1983) 1009 Consecutive carotid endarterectomies using local anesthesia. EEG and selective shunting with the Pruitt Inahara carotid shunt. Contemp Surg 23: 49–58

Author's address:
Univ.-Prof. Dr. G. W. Hagmüller
Chirurgische Abt.
Wilhelminenspital der Stadt Wien
Montleartstr. 37
A-1160 Wien, Austria

Intraoperative angiography in carotid surgery

K. Balzer[1], J. D. Gruss[2], W. Lang[3]

Department for Vascular Surgery[1] (Head: Dr. K. Balzer) Evangelisches Krankenhaus Muelheim an der Ruhr, Department for Vascular Surgery[2] (Head: Prof. Dr. J. D. Gruss) Kurhessisches Diakonissenhaus Kassel and the Department for Vascular Surgery University of Erlangen[3] (Germany)

Introduction

As the NASCET and ECST show carotid endarterectomy has proved to be highly effective in the prevention of ischemic stroke. For that, a stroke rate of less than 3 % and a death rate of less than 1 % is necessary. This makes intraoperative assessment of the completed operation mandatory. For this, intraoperative angiography is the most suitable, but some authors are claiming instead of an angiogramm that the angioscopy is more suitable.

Patients and methods

We investigated intraoperative findings by angiography and angioscopy in three vascular surgical centers. In Kassel 1187 carotid endarterectomies and 964 angiograms were performed between 1986 and 1994.

In Mülheim over the last 5 years, in a total of 2476 carotid operations, angioscopy was the method of choice. An angiogram was only done in cases in which angioscopy could not be performed or showed suspicious findings. That was necessary only in 87 operations, 83 eversion endarterectomies, and 4 conventional endarterectomies. Neither an angioscopy nor an angiography was performed in 234 patients because of clear intraoperative findings.

A prospective study showing the importance of intraoperative quality control at the University of Erlangen with 245 intraoperative angiograms on 274 carotid operations was done in the last two years.

The technique for intraoperative angiography was nearly the same in all of the three centers: Before closing the arteriotomy the angiographic cannula is introduced directly or via the upper thyreoideal artery. The cannula is placed under direct view over the central intimal step into the common carotid artery. This procedure prevents direct damaging of the desobliterated arterial segment and a possible dissection of the central intima. After restoring the flow through the external and internal carotid artery, 10 ml of contrast medium were injected by the surgeon and the carotid artery system was visualized on the monitor in different planes. The result of the angiography can be documented by a simple photograph; however, a radiogram can also be taken. After withdrawing the cannula, the thyreoideal artery was closed simply with two metal clips or the puncture stopped bleeding spontaneously. If routinely done, intraoperative angiography does not take more than five minutes.

The same is true for intraoperative angioscopy: After withdrawing the occasionally implanted shunt and before final closure of the arteriotomy, a 2.2 or 2.4 mm angioscope is introduced through the remaining opening. The peripheral lumen, the distal intimal step, the endarterectomized part of the internal carotid artery and the central part of the external carotid artery are inspected on the monitor. In eversion endarterectomy this procedure should be done before the first stay suture is performed. Thus, the possibility for a renewed eversion is open. Care must be taken not to overestimate small intimal flaps or adherent thrombi. When starting with this method it was difficult to interpret the magnification effect correctly and for that, in all of the three centers in a couple of cases, intraoperative angioscopy was combined with additional intraoperative angiography. In 11 % of the cases in Erlangen and 19 % in the cases in Kassel but only in 3.9 % of the operations in Mülheim neither an angiogram nor an angioscopy were performed. Most of these in Kassel were from early cases thinking a contralateral occlusion could be a contraindication for the use of the dye injection. In Erlangen most of the non-inspected cases were due to technical problems.

Results

Adverse events related to the intraoperative angiography were found due to an allergic reaction in 3 of 245 cases (= 1 %) in Erlangen, in 1 of 87 cases (= 1.3 %) in Mülheim but in none of the 964 angiograms in Kassel, from which 79 were interpreted as abnormal, indicating the surgical revision (8.2 %). Nearly the same amount was found in the cases from Erlangen. There were 20 % pathological findings, which is the same as in the beginning of

Table 1. Intraoperative angiography in carotid surgery

Vascular centers	normal	pathol.
Erlangen	77 %	23 %
Kassel 1986	80 %	20 %
Kassel 1990	94 %	6 %
Kassel 1994	95 %	5 %
Mülheim (Ruhr)	82 %	18 %

Table 2. Intraoperative angiography in carotid surgery

		Literature (n)	pathol.	revis.	interna
Anderson	1978	131	5.3 %	5.3 %	2.5 %
Scottgen	1982	107	52.3 %	16.8 %	11.2 %
Jernigan	1984	603		2.4 %	
Del Bosque	1989	106	17.9 %	8.5 %	6.6 %
Donaldson	1992	410	17.3 %	16.1 %	10.2 %
Roon	1992	535	2.1 %		

the series in Kassel. In the next years in Kassel it was possible to reduce the revision rate by paying more attention to special technical aspects, in particular a meticulous endarterectomy with an appropriate distal endpoint using tacking sutures; however even after a short period of time, less than a 3 % revision rate in 1992 in 1994 again more than 4 % of revisions were necessary. This rate is similar in Erlangen concerning the internal carotid artery (3.7 %) and in Mülheim (3.8 %), and it is also published in the literature by many investigators, ranging from 2.1 to 52.3 % pathological findings (Table 2).

Examples

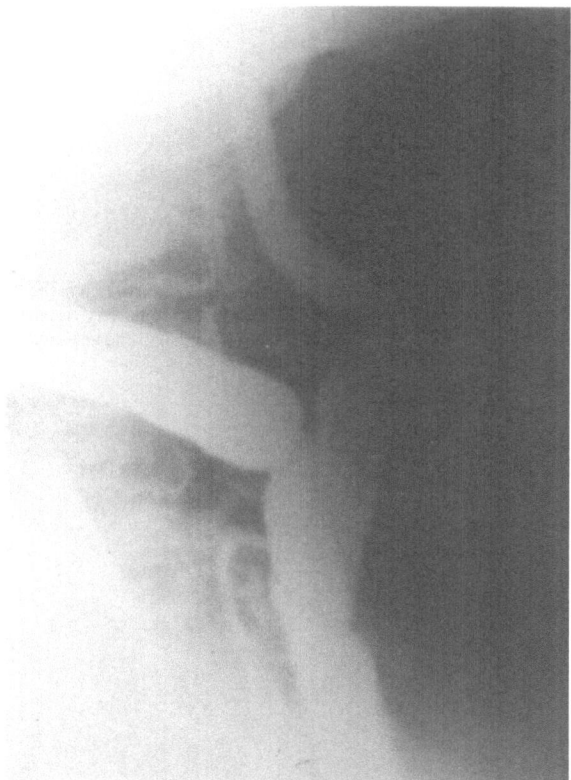

Fig. 1. Kinking phenomenon after unsufficient shortening of the internal carotid artery.

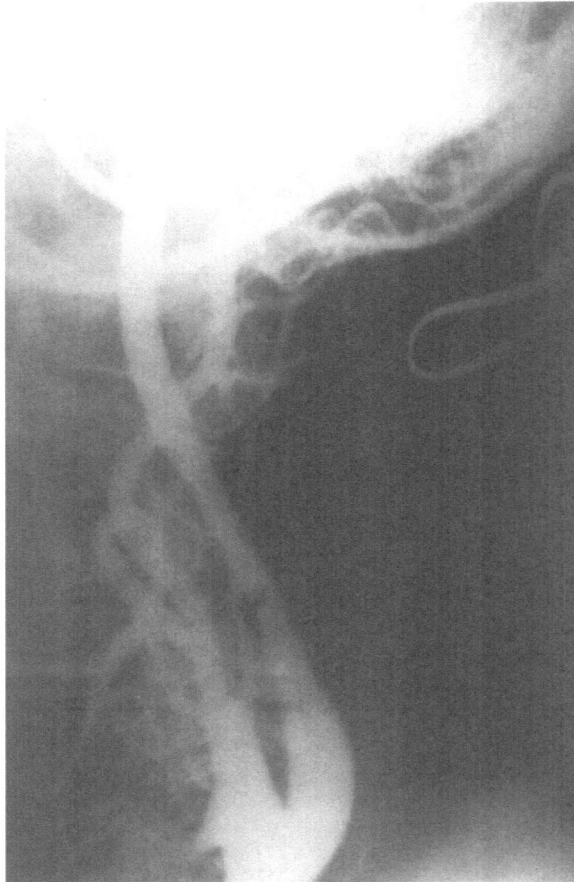

Fig. 2a, b. Intimal flap in the internal carotid artery visualized by angiography and angioscopy.

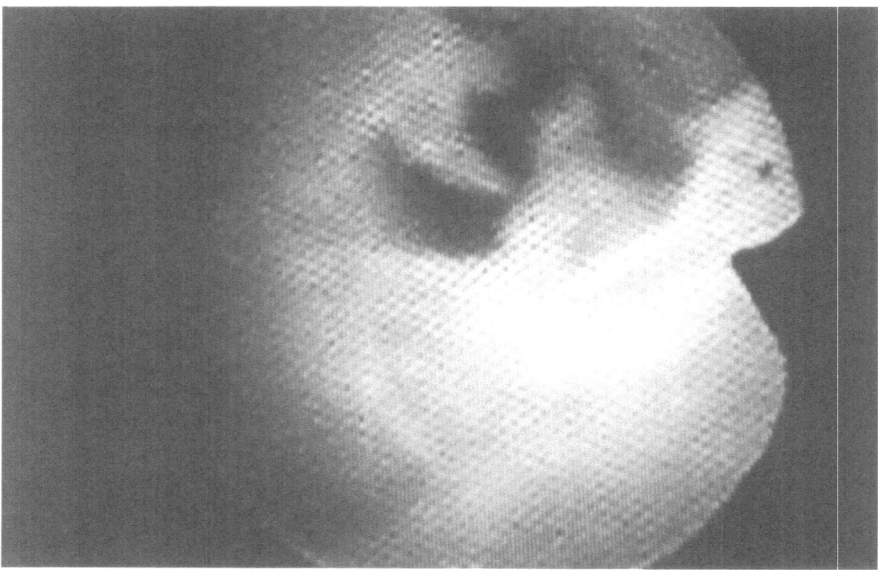

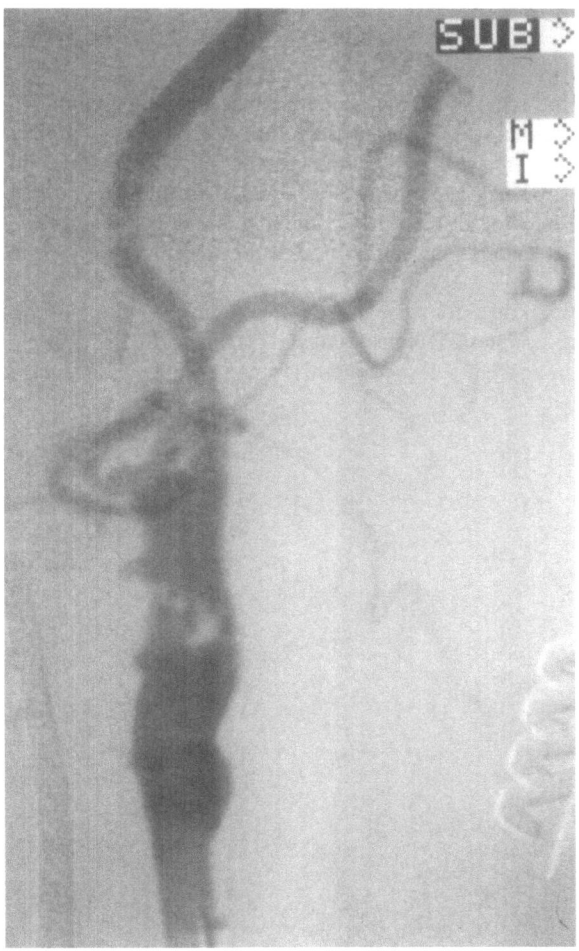

Fig. 3. Stenosis after patch plasty of the internal carotid artery which must lead to a subsequent thrombosis.

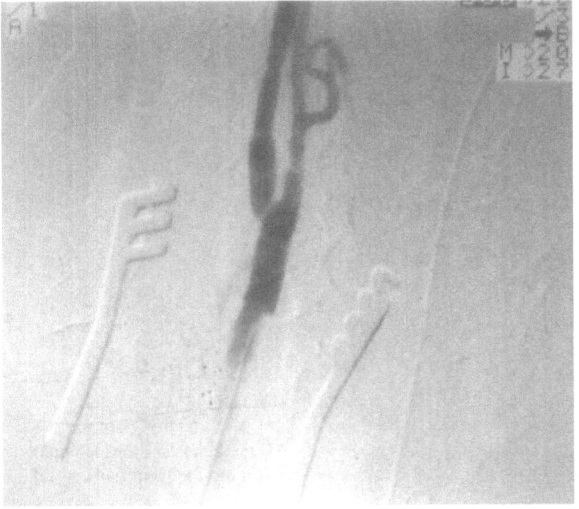

Fib. 4. Stenosis after replanting the internal carotid artery in eversion endarterectomy.

Discussion

Intraoperative angiography and intraoperative angioscopy are both suitable methods to detect technical abnormalities after carotid reconstruction. Intraoperative angiography has the advantage that vascular surgeons are familiar with the angiographic technique and the interpretation of angiograms. The disadvantages are the need to inject a contrast medium and the use of x-rays. On the other hand, intraoperative angioscopy requires a longer learning period because the magnifying effect makes the interpretation of the different findings difficult.

The advantages are that there is no need for a contrast medium nor for x-ray exposure. Undoubtedly, angioscopy is more traumatic and may damage mechanically the thrombendarterectomized carotid segment as well as the peripheral intima. Another disadvantage

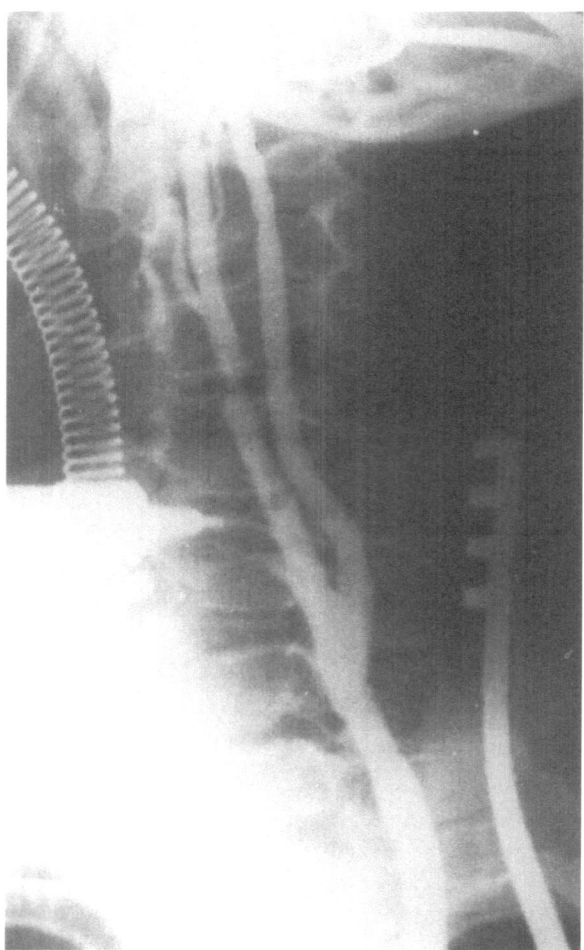

Fig. 5. Stenosis of the incomplete desobliterated external carotid artery.

is the prolongation of the clamping time which might be important in cases with associated contralateral carotid or vertebral occlusions. The number of technical errors which need correction reported in the literature are in the same range around 6 %. Kinney et al. using duplex scanning and pulsed Doppler spectral analysis alone or in combination with intra-operative angiography published a revision rate of 5.6 %. Perioperative morbidity (30 days) was similar in patients with normal and mildly abnormal completion studies. There were 1.3 % permanent and 2.6 % temporary neurological deficits. In the follow-up period the incidence of cases in which the lumen were reduced by >50 % stenoses or occlusion was increased in patients with residual flow abnormalities. Patients with normal intra-operative flow-studies had significantly lower rates of late ipsilateral stroke compared with the remaining patient group. During the mean 30 months follow-up interval, the incidence of late stroke was increased in patients with internal carotid artery restenosis or occlusion (3/35) compared with patients without recurrent stenoses (3/424).

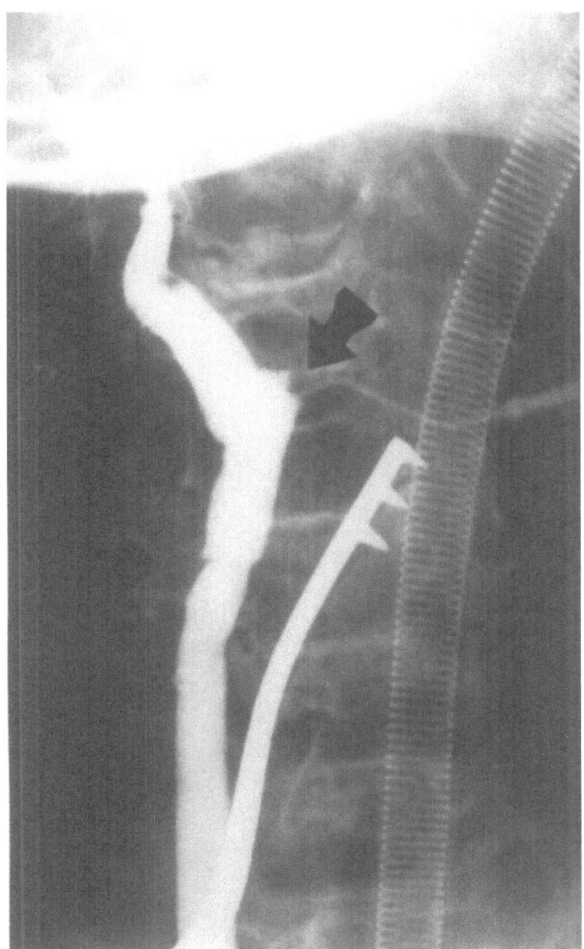

Fig. 6. Occlusion of the external carotid artery.

Conclusions

Our results strongly support our decision to continue routinely visualizing all carotid endarterectomies with an intraoperative quality control using either angiography or angioscopy. Confirmation of a normal repair at operation affords the best possibility of minimizing ischemic neurologic events and pathologic restenosis after carotid endarterectomy.

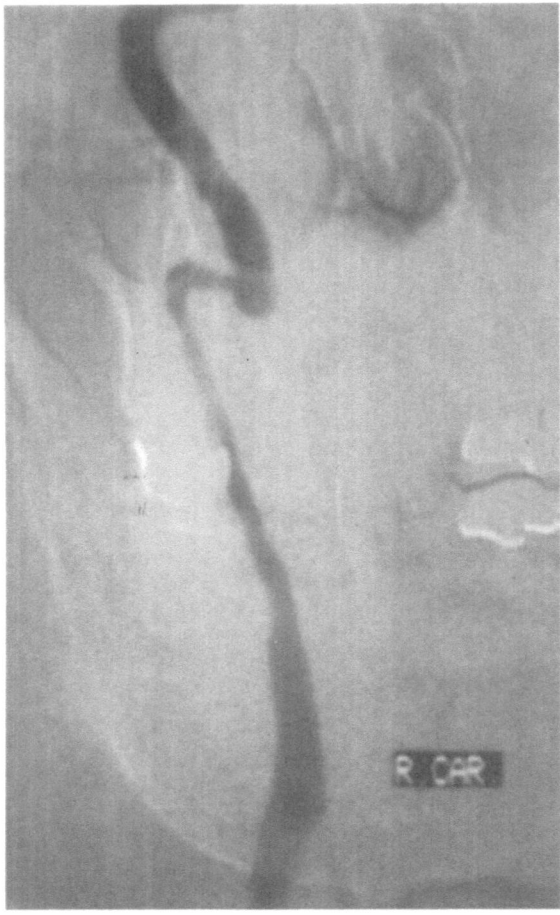

Fig. 7. Incomplete thrombosis of the internal carotid artery.

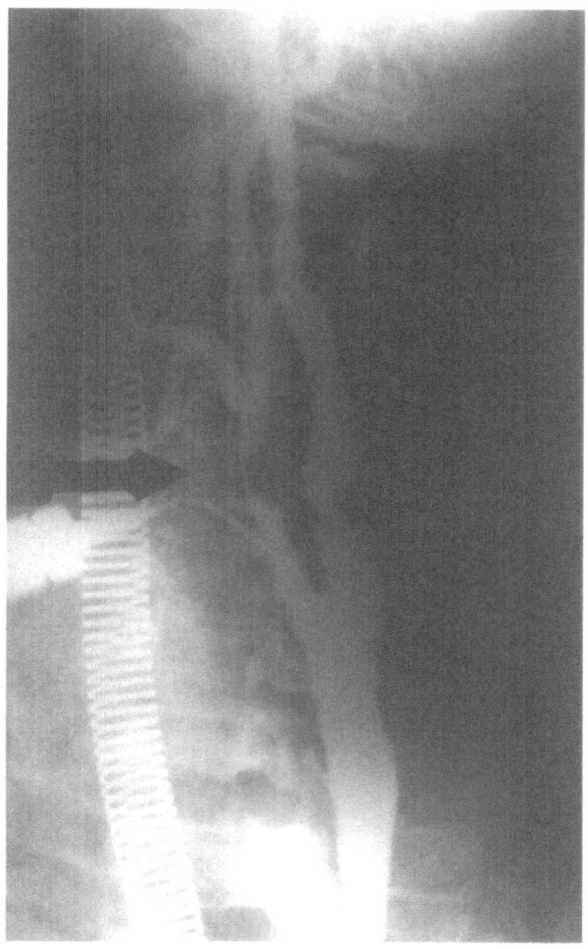

Fig. 8. Stenosis of internal and external carotid artery.

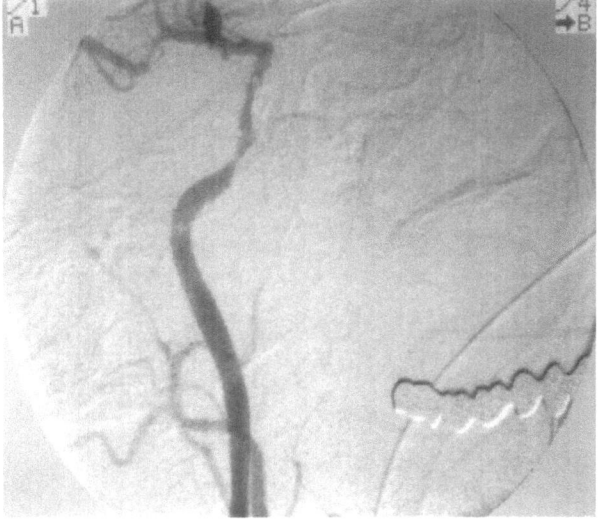

Fig. 9. Intracranial stenosis of the carotid syphon.

References

1. Donaldson MC, Ivarsson BL, Mannick JA, Whittmore AD (1993) Impact of completion angiography on operative conduct and results of carotid endarterectomy. Ann Surg 217: 682–687
2. European Carotid Surgery Trialists' Collaborative Group (1991) MRC European Carotid Surgery Trial: interim results for symptomatic patients with severe (70–99 %) or with mild (0–29 %) carotid stenosis. Lancet 337: 1235–1243
3. Gruss JD (1996) Intraoperative completion angiography and angioscopy in carotid artery surgery. In: Caplan LR, Shifrin E, Nocolaides AN, Moore WS (eds): Cerebrovascular Ischaemia. Investigation and Management. Med Orion Publishing Company. London Los Angeles Nicosia: 255–262
4. Hoff C, de Gier P, Buth J (1994) Intraoperative duplex monitoring of the carotid bifurcation for the detection of technical defects. Eur J Vasc Surg 8: 441–447
5. Kinney EV, Seabrock GR, Kinney LY, Bandyk DF (1993) The importance of intraoperative detection of residual flow abnormalities after carotid artery endarterectomy. J Vasc Surg 17: 912–923
6. Lohr JM, Albers B, Roat TW, Byrne MP, Roedersheimer LR, Piercefield GG (1995) Effects of completion angiography on the outcome of carotid endarterectomy. Cardiovascular Surgery. 3: 299–305
7. North American Symptomatic Carotid Endarterectomy Trial Collaborators (1991) Beneficial effect of carotid endarterectomy in symptomatic patients with highgrade carotid stenosis. N Engl J Med 325: 446–453
8. Raithel D (1993) Intraoperative angioscopy after carotid endarterectomy. J Mal Vasc 18: 258–261
9. Roon AJ, Hoogerwerf D (1992) Intraoperative arteriography and carotid surgery. J Vasc Surg 16: 239–243

Author's address:
Klaus Balzer, MD.
Chefarzt der Gefäßchirurgischen Klinik
am Evangelischen Krankenhaus
Wertgasse 30
45468 Mülheim an der Ruhr, Germany

Intraoperative electroencephalography (EEG) monitoring and clinical outcome in carotid surgery

W. Sandmann

Department of Vascular Surgery and Kidney Transplantation, University of Düsseldorf

These is no doubt, that electroencephalography can show variations during carotid end-arterectomy before and after clamping. Many authors, especially in the English speaking literature have done a lot of work to prove that it is worthwhile to monitor the patients during carotid endarterectomy; however, the native EEG may be difficult to interpret at least for vascular surgeons while a spectral arrangement might be easier to interpret.

It has been shown several years ago by McKay and associates in Birmingham, Albama, that if you compare EEG monitoring and regional cerebral blood flow measurement then the largest changes in the group with the least regional blood flow are found. However, looking for complications afterwards especially in the group with very low flows, despite the fact that there were significant changes in EEG monitoring, there was an uneventful clinical outcome. So the problem is that those changes observed during surgery do not necessarily cause a bad clinical outcome, and they are probably only a rough guidance to which cases selective shunting should be used, because this is all about EEG in those patients. Another problem is that regional blood flow does not have a very clear relation to the internal carotid artery stump pressure, a method which was used several years ago to find out which patients might need a shunt and which do not; if one sees the squares and the crosses and the points pointing hallothane, enflurane, and influrane anaesthesia one may realize that there is a great variation of regional cerebral blood flow (RCBF) and internal carotid stump pressure. Since RCBF is only poorly related to clinical outcome, the surgeon is lost in a chaotic amount of those values.

In our prospective study, there were 503 patients in which at random shunting had been performed or avoided. Just to have a quick look, there were 250 patients planned for shunting out of which 35 could not be shunted for technical reasons, while 253 were planned without shunting and 10 of those had to be shunted because of significant changes either in EEG or evoked potentials. In summary, what came out of this study in one aspect was if significant changes occur during clamping and they do not only occur after 3 or 5 minutes, they can occur even after 20 or 30 minutes of clamping if such a long time is needed to reconstruct the artery and a shunt is not inserted very quickly which was not done at that time, then a high perioperative stroke rate is observed: 42 % out of these 19 patients, while in those with normal EEG and/or evoked potentials, the perioperative stroke rate was very low 1.2 %. The postoperative stroke rate showed some relations, too, but these were not significant. Significant were those occuring during surgery.

Using as an example a comparison between evoked potentials and EEG out of a subset of this study, the preoperative clinical findings were correlated with the electroencephalogram or the SEP's before clamping of the internal carotid artery. With EEG there were about 6 % of the patients in which it was not possible to evaluate the EEG because there were so many electrical disturbances. This is one of the disadvantages of this type of recording. The same at that time was true for recording of the evoked potentials, but it could be that in one patient the evoked potentials were not evaluable while the EEG was wonderful and vice versa.

It was also noted that in those patients which had experienced a stroke prior to surgery, the most reversable and irreversable changes in the EEG were registered and the same was true for evoked potentials. In patients who were asymptomatic or had non-hemispheric symptoms, only a few changes were noticed, and most of these had normal recordings before clamping.

The postoperative clinical findings related to the intraoperative recordings of the EEG and SEP showed some amazing results. The positive predictive value coming from irreversable changes determing clinical outcome for EEG was only 50 % while for evoked potentials it was 100 %. The positive predictive value for those who had a normal EEG before, during, and after clamping time, the positive predictive value that they will not develop neurological ischaemic deficit was 97 % with the EEG and 96 % for the evoked potentials. The problem is that with these monitoring devices good methods to show some significant changes during surgery to make us alert are available, but whether the patient will awake without or with a neurological problem is not known. However, if with SEP monitoring there is a significant change, and this will be found at the end of surgery as well, then it is certain that the patient will awake with a neurological problem, but with EEG it is clearly not the same.

In conclusion, I am not so much fond today of EEG monitoring because evoked potentials tend to give us simpler possibilities to evaluate the patient during surgery. During carotid surgery all of these various parameters should be monitored and we think that either SEP or EEG is mandatory in carotid endarterectomy. It is difficult to understand why there are still many surgeons who do not evaluate brain function during surgery of vessels which supply the blood to the brain. Perfusion ischaemia must be detected by one or the other methods and if it occurs, prophylactic measures to protect the patient against stroke must be taken. Under these circumstances, unrestricted flow and anatomical reconstruction can be achieved without hurrying through the procedure.

References

available from the author

Author's address:
W. Sandmann, MD
Department of Vascular Surgery and
Kidney Transplantation
University of Düsseldorf
Moorenstr. 5
40225 Düsseldorf, Germany

ICBP in comparison to the intraoperative EEG monitoring

H. Loeprecht

Department of Thoracic and Vascular Surgery, Central Hospital, Augsburg

We have already heard something about EEG monitoring this morning as well as this afternoon by Prof. Sandmann. I would like to discuss with you our experience using the EEG as intra-operative control method. A prospective evaluation performed 10 years ago related to the fact that up until this time only back pressure measurements for intra-operative monitoring purposes were performed as proposed by Wesley Moore. At this stage, it was considered whether perhaps one could perform selective shunting when using the ICBP as monitoring, but as the Circle of Willis is not always complete, but very often is interrupted or numerous variations may exist, this did not appear reliable as the only criterium for judging the necessity of a shunt. The back pressure is not only dependent on the contralateral stenosis, but frequently on the vascular arrangement of the Circle of Willis.

Presently, an EEG Trend Analyser with a print-out of the curves as well as the power spectrum is being used. Normally, the vast quantities of data from the regular EEG need to be analysed by a neurologist, a completely impractical situation in an operating theater. The EEG Trend Analyser performs a fast summation analysis and retrospectively the frequency, the shifting of frequencies, as well as the amplitude changes can still be seen.

Here is an example of the print-out of the data: the power of the entire curve and also of the singular frequency bands can be seen. This is a normal curve of a 2 channel EEG, a curve which can also be correctly interpreted by the surgeon and give an idea of how the clamping has affected the cerebral perfusion. The criteria for a pathological EEG is a power reduction of more than 20 % in the ipsilateral channel or a visibly recognizable frequency shift of the ipsilateral side.

This is a presentation of the the clamping period, the 1st clamping period, recovery of the trace after insertion of a shunt, then removal of the shunt, and consequent clamping with a recurrent amplitude reduction. Back pressure, as mentioned this morning by Mr. Moore, has a threshold of perhaps 20 mmHg, but I consider this threshold to be too low. Consequently, generally accepted at least in Germany is to use a figure of 50 mmHg; however, beyond this threshold for back-pressure, it is considered absolutely necessary to introduce a shunt – or perhaps this is also disputable. The results from this prospective study which included 150 patients incorporating 109 men and 41 women with a mean age of 66 years will be presented.

The neurological status of the patients requiring an endarterectomy of the carotid was an asymptomatic (stage I) disease in 44 patients, stage II disease in 58 patients, and a progressive stroke in 8 patients. 40 % of patients had suffered a fulminant stroke and were in a stable condition at the time of surgery.

A correlation between the stump pressure and the degree of stenosis as it was noticed with the SEP curve mentioned in an earlier presentation today could not be established in these trials. Only in the presence of an extremely high-grade stenosis did the stump pressure increase correspondingly, probably ascribable to the better developed collateral circulation.

Using the Trend Analyser 150 EEG recordings were assessed and 37 pathological recordings were noticed. These were all related to the stage of the disease. As further demonstrated here, no great variation was noticed, and the difference was not statistically significant. This corresponds to the data shown by Dr. Imperato that there is a need for shunting when using the EEG method in 25 % of cases.

In an intermediate evaluation of these series using a threshold of 50 mmHg as the critical point for shunt insertion, only a sensitivity of 67 % and a specificity of 61 % were recorded. When a lower threshold of 20 to 30 mmHg was used, the specificity is high and the sensitivity zero, this being the reason for mentioning the variation of accepted thresholds earlier. In this patient group of 150 patients, 5 presented with a newly acquired post-operative neurological deficit of which the EEG identified 4 abnormal traces. In all these patients the back-pressure was very high: not 20 mmHg, but varying between 45 and 80 mmHg. The clinical stage the patient was in when surgery was performed was also assessed. 50 % had ulcerated plaque intra-operatively. Three patients had a temporary neurological deficit post-operatively and 2 patients suffered a permanent neurological deficit. The additional problem of the stenotic contralateral internal carotid artery in this series showed that in contralateral stenosis a slight increase of pathological EEG findings was observed, but contrary to expectations the back pressure was slightly, but not significantly different in the presence of contralateral occlusion. Neither in the EEG trace nor in the back pressure measurements was there a statistically significant difference.

Calculating sensitivity and specificity values from this data, sensitivity of the back pressure was only 40 % even when applying 50 mmHg as a threshold. The EEG's sensitivity was as high as 80 %; the specificity was 77 % and for back pressure measurements 54 %. The same figures applied to the positive predictive value.

In summary, one could say that back pressure gives an accurate indication of the efficiency of the collateral circulation via the Circle of Willis, but does not supply any information about the effectiveness of cerebral perfusion. Additionally, the EEG trend analyser method for monitoring is more reliable, but is not accurate enough to set the indication for selective shunting. The aim was to establish whether the EEG trace analyser can be used as a selection criterium for selective shunting, but from the mentioned results the answer to this question is clearly negative. For this reason, a shunt is routinely inserted for all the carotid endarterectomies that are performed at our clinic.

References

available from the author

Author's address:
H. Loeprecht, MD
Department of Thoracic and Vascular Surgery
Central Hospital Augsburg
Steglinstr. 1
86156 Augsburg, Germany

Internal carotid back pressure versus somatosensory evoked potentials to determine shunt requirement

H. Schweiger, R. Rümenapf

Dep. of Vascular Surgery (Prof. Dr. H. Schweiger), Rhönklinikum, Bad Neustadt

The use of a temporary shunt in carotid artery reconstructions remains controversial. A variety of monitoring methods have been proposed to find out those patients who do not tolerate clamping of the internal carotid artery even for a few minutes. In recent years somatosensory evoked potentials (SEP) were shown to be a very accurate method to detect hemispheric cerebral ischemia. However, an experienced assistance is neccessary for this method, it may be time consuming, and it may not be available in smaller institutions.

In contrast to SEP recording which judges the function of the brain, carotid artery stump pressure (CSP) measurements estimate the perfusion pressure of the ipsilateral hemisphere when the internal carotid artery is clamped. As this method is inexpensive, almost ubiquitously available and easy to perform, it is hitherto widely used for estimating cerebral blood flow to brain areas supplied by the clamped artery. However, there is little information about the sensitivity and specificity of CSP in detecting cerebral ischemia. Therefore, we compared the results of SEP recording with those of CSP measurements.

Patients and methods

During internal carotid artery reconstructions, both CSP and SEP were recorded. The method of SEP monitoring is described elsewere. After cross-clamping of the common and external carotid artery a 20-gauge needle connected by a catheter to an electromechanical pressure transducer was inserted into the common or internal carotid artery. The mean carotid stump pressure was measured for 1 to 2 min.

Anesthesia was finished after wound closure, and all patients were extubated in the operating room to obtain immediate information about their neurologic status before transport to the recovery room.

There were 363 patients, 69.9 % were male. The mean age of the patients was 68.7 years. The indication for operation was a transient ischemic attack or an amaurosis fugax in 139 cases, a completed stroke with minimal or moderate residual neurologic deficit in 97 cases, and 127 patients were asymptomatic.

Results and discussion

During 325 carotid endarteriectomies, the SEP amplitudes were always identified, and a shunt was never used. The mean CSP in these cases was 49.7 mm Hg. No patient had a new neurologic deficit after extubation. In some cases, a marked decrease of SEP amplitude was recorded during the clamping period, but the amplitudes were always identified. None of these patients was operated with the use of a shunt, and no patient showed a deficit.

In contrast, complete loss of SEP-amplitude occurred in 38 cases. The mean CSP measured after clamping was 20.7 mm Hg (range: 10 – 41 mm Hg). Six patients were operated without the use of an indwelling shunt, and three of them showed a transient neurologic deficit. In 32 cases, a shunt was used following disappearance of SEP amplitudes, and seven experienced a deficit.

There was a close correlation between CSP and the frequency of loss of SEP amplitudes during clamping (Table 1). For example, seven patients had a CSP of 15 mm Hg or lower, and all had loss of SEP-amplitude after clamping. When the CSP was higher than 35 mm Hg (232 patients) a complete loss of SEP-amplitude was observed in one case only.

The accuracy of CSP in detecting cerebral ischemia (according to SEP criteria) is shown in Table 2. A sensitivity of 100 % is achieved, when a CSP of 50 mm Hg or lower is regarded as critical. However, the specificity is quiet low (40 %) and, when this limit is used an unneccessary shunting will occur in as much as 50 % of the cases. On the other hand, when a lower limit is used the sensitivity of this method will decrease.

The data presented indicate that CSP measurement shows a good correlation with SEP results. CSP may be regarded as a reliable predictor of collateral cerebral perfusion pres-

Table 1. Relation between CSP and loss of SEP

CSP (mm Hg)	N	Los of SEP-amplitude	
		N	%
10 – 15	7	7	100
16 – 20	27	17	63
21 – 25	30	6	20
26 – 30	29	5	17
31 – 35	27	2	7
36 – 40	32	0	0
41 – 45	27	1	4
46 – 110	174	0	0

Table 2. Sensitivity and specificity of CSP in detecting clamping ischemia and the assumed rate of unnecessary shunting according to SEP criteria.

CSP-range (mm Hg)	Sensitivity (%)	Specificity (%)	Unnecessary shunting (%)
0 – 25	79	90	9
0 – 30	92	82	19
0 – 50	100	40	50

sure. Since CSP does not estimate brain function it is an indirect predictor of cerebral ischemia. Despite high CSP values, a much lower perfusion pressure may be present in postocclusive intracerebral areas. This may lead to severe brain damage and, of course, cannot be detected by CSP measurement.

In general, CSP measurement is a valuable method to estimate hemispheric perfusion and, indirectly, brain function. In some few cases, however, cerebral ischemia is present despite high CSP. To our opinion, monitoring brain function by SEP is the better option.

References

available from the author

Author's address:
Prof. Dr. H. Schweiger
Abteilung für Gefäßchirurgie
Herz- und Gefäßklinik
Rhönklinikum
Salzburger Leite 1
97616 Bad Neustadt, Germany

Intraoperative monitoring during carotid endarterectomy: SEP versus EEG monitoring

E. Fava, F. Lang, P. L. Vandone[1], E. Bortolani[2], M. Schieppati[3]

Istituto di Neurochirurgia, [1]Istituto di Chirurgia Generale e Cardiovascolare, [2]Cattedra di Chirurgia Generale, Università di Milano, Milan; [3]Istituto di Fisiologia Umana, Università di Genova, Genoa; Italy.

Introduction

Carotid endarterectomy is a controversial surgery from several points of view, and the possibility of intraoperative stroke due to temporary carotid occlusion still raises great concern. Many techniques have been developed to reduce this risk since the first carotid endarterectomy was performed by De Bakey in 1953. The main goal of brain monitoring in carotid surgery is to detect patients at risk of brain ischemia on carotid occlusion and to give indication for temporary shunt.

Recording electrical activity of the brain can be used as a monitor of cerebral perfusion in anesthetized patients, owing to its relationship with cerebral blood flow (CBF) (16). In acute reductions of CBF, there is a wide range of flow values corresponding to what is known as ischemic penumbra, wherein blood flow is below that required for normal electrical activity, but is still adequate for maintaining viable neural tissue. This condition of functional suppression of the electrical activity of the brain was demonstrated to be reversible (1, 2, 3) even if maintained for a period of up to 6 h (9). On these grounds, it is evident how neurophysiological techniques enable us to detect early warnings of reduced cerebral perfusion before a permanent damage ensues, and to obtain some clues about the success of the maneuvers adopted to reverse an impending brain ischemia. Ordinary electroencephalogram (EEG) was the first technique that was extensively used in patients operated on under general anesthesia, and Somatosensory Evoked Potentials (SEP) were introduced in the 1980s. Both methods are now widely accepted as sensitive, reliable and safe in this application, and they can easily be employed throughout the surgery.

EEG and SEP recording

Our experience is based on recording of both EEG and cortical SEP in all carotid endarterectomies performed under general anesthesia with or without shunt, in the last 8 years in the Department of General and Cardiovascular Surgery of the University of Milano. The techniques used during all operations are briefly recalled hereafter: seven to eight channels of unprocessed digital EEG were recorded over both hemispheres; cortical SEP after median nerve stimulation were collected from parietal scalp electrodes at the C3/C4 positions in the International 10/20 System (8), with the contralateral electrode referred to the ipsilateral one. EEG was continuously recorded, while SEP were obtained approximately every 50 s, since 200 post-stimulus epochs were averaged at a stimulation frequency of 4 Hz. The recordings of EEG and SEP from the non-operated side served as the control, in order to discern between the effects of surgical manipulation which are mostly unilateral and general effects due to changes in anesthesia or arterial blood pressure which are mostly bilateral. Hook-shaped subcutaneous needle electrodes were used both for recording brain electrical activity and for stimulating the median nerve at the wrist.

The operations were performed under general anesthesia with Isoflurane and nitrous oxide. Brain monitoring started after induction of anesthesia, when the patient was still supine, i.e., before the head was turned in the surgical position, and it ended when the patient was awakened by the anesthesiologist. Tolerance to carotid occlusion was tested by observation of EEG and SEP in a 2-min period following carotid clamping, before arteriotomy. Whenever electrical abnormalities appeared, an attempt was made to reverse them by inducing a slight hypertension. A temporary shunt was used in case of failure of this attempt.

We considered signs of impending brain ischemia due to carotid clamping to be the sudden occurrence of EEG slow waves or the sudden reduction of the amplitude of the waves, and the reduced amplitude or increased latency of N20/P25 complex of SEP (see Fig. 1). On carotid occlusion, EEG changes became evident earlier than SEP changes, since at best a 50-s interval had to elapse before a post-clamp SEP could be analyzed.

Early findings

At the beginning of our experience, the surgeon's bias against unnecessary use of shunts led to its use only in patients showing alarming changes in both EEG and cortical SEP. The retrospective analysis of the data led us to quantify SEP changes, in order to assess the safety of this procedure and to reduce the inter-observer variability. In fact, while alarming EEG changes due to acute cerebral ischemia have been described by many authors (4, 5, 10), less agreement existed as far as SEP in humans were concerned (7, 11, 12, 14). In 1992, we published our first series of 151 operations in which indication for temporary shunt was provided by both EEG and SEP (6). Acute worsening of SEP appeared as a reduction of amplitude and/or an increase of latency that first affected P25 wave (Fig. 1, bottom right), then also N20. We then used clamp-related changes of latency and amplitude of P25 wave to build up a Need-for-Shunt Index (NSI):

$$\frac{\text{post-clamp P25 latency}}{\text{pre-clamp P25 latency}} - \frac{\text{post-clamp P25 amplitude}}{\text{pre-clamp P25 amplitude}}$$

It is evident how in absence of SEP changes, NSI equals zero, while the worse is SEP after carotid occlusion the higher is NSI. We therefore defined a threshold value beyond which shunt was mandatory (NSI = 0.5). In that series shunt rate was 10.6 %, while if EEG criterion alone would have been used shunt rate would have been 20.5 %. In fact, major abnormalities were induced twice as frequently on EEG than on SEP by carotid occlusion. We had no neurological complication in the patients who developed EEG changes alone, but did not receive shunting on the basis of SEP behavior. Among shunted patients, two (12.5 %) awoke with a new neurological deficit. Among non-shunted patients, one (0.7 %) developed a stroke after several tens of minutes of uneventful carotid clamping, when SEP suddenly disappeared with almost unmodified EEG.

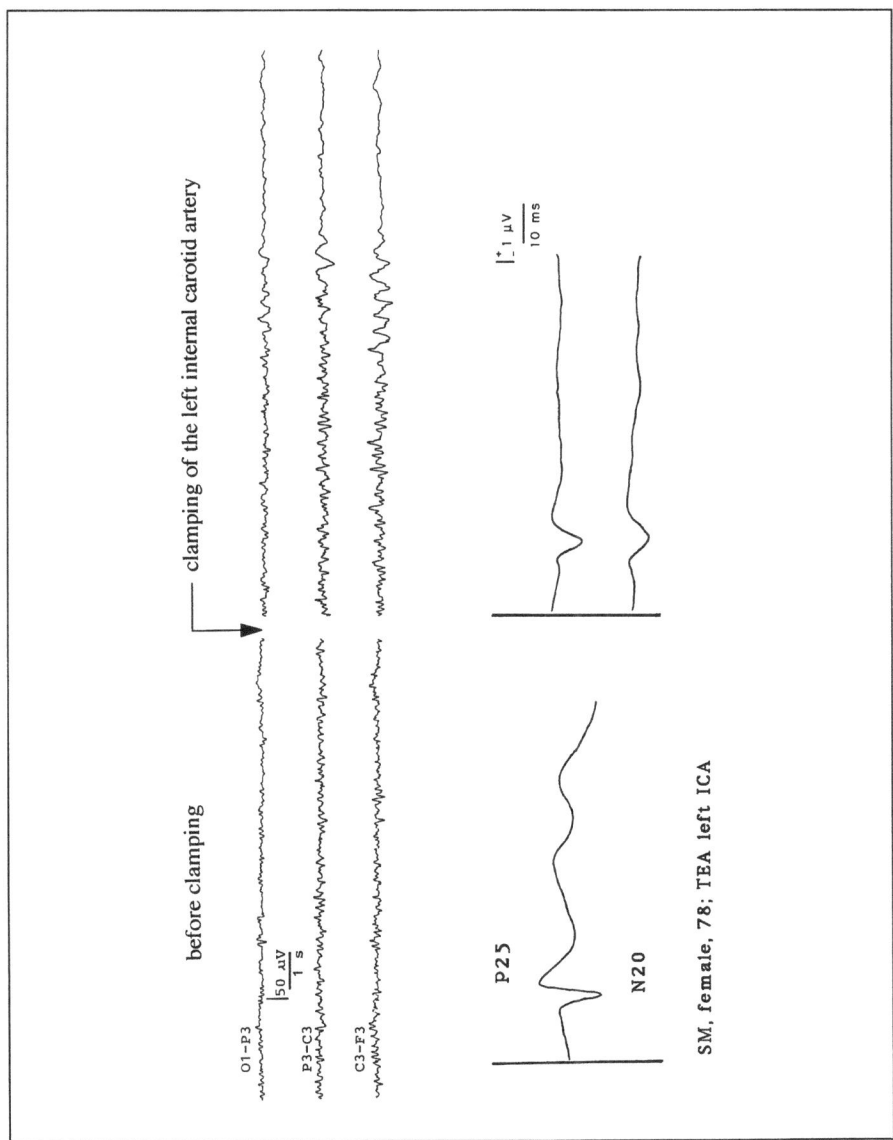

Fig. 1. Samples of EEG (top) and SEP (bottom) before (left) and after (right) carotid occlusion in a patient who developed signs of brain ischemia due to left carotid clamping and subsequently received temporary shunt. Immediately after carotid occlusion EEG (top right) showed slow waves and in a few seconds its amplitude was severely depressed; the first two post-clamp SEPs showed progressive delay and decrement of P25 and N20 peaks.

New findings

In the last series of operations, we have been using SEP and NSI prospectively, for allotting patients to shunt or no-shunt groups, even if EEG has always been recorded. A total of 127 operations have been performed in the last 4 years, with shunt rate of 6.3 % (eight patients). One patient of the non-shunted group and one patient who received the shunt developed intraoperative neurological complications (1.6 % overall morbidity; 12.5 % in patients with shunt; 0.8 % in patients without shunt). The non-shunted patient had received no shunt despite that her NSI was as high as 0.85 due to surgical troubles that prevented the surgeon to even perform endarterectomy (the operated carotid artery had to be ligated at the end of the operation, and the patient was comatose and hemiplegic after surgery). The other patient had NSI of 0.73 and a Pruitt shunt was inserted. Since it allowed just a minor recovery of EEG and SEP, the surgeon replaced it with a Javid shunt of larger diameter, which enabled a good recovery of SEP and EEG. The patient awoke with arm paresis that cleared in a few hours.

The values of NSI in patients operated on without temporary shunt ranged from -0.8 to 0.571 (mean 0.039; SD 0.227), while in shunted patients the values ranged from 0.42 to 0.91 (mean 0.682; SD 0.157). The two groups are significantly different ($p < 0.0001$). The single patient who was shunted despite his NSI value of 0.42 was done by the surgeon since his EEG showed "alarming" signs of impending brain ischemia. We believe that in this case SEP did not show striking worsening after carotid occlusion since it was pathological over both hemispheres even before carotid occlusion, due to previous cerebrovascular accidents. It remains to be assessed whether the NSI methods should be used or not in such patients.

Therefore, we conclude on the basis of the last 127 operations analyzed that a threshold NSI value of 0.5 is a good predictor for the need for shunt.

Conclusions

We have a strong bias in favor of the SEP as a means of identifying patients in need of shunt during carotid endarterectomy, for several reasons. First, they test the entire somatosensory pathway including the subcortical regions, where critical changes in blood flow may develop that are not detected by EEG (15). Second, they are more resistant than EEG to reduced cerebral blood flow (CBF) and to pharmacological depression (13). Third, they can be easily recorded from just two electrodes on the head of the patient. Fourth, their acute changes can be easily quantified by a descriptor like the NSI. EEG mostly reflects cortical activity, it is deeply modified by anesthetics, and by reduced CBF at a level that is higher than for SEP (13); it requires at least 10 electrodes on the head of the patient.

Of course, we do not believe that EEG must be abandoned, mostly because it has the property of changing earlier than SEP after any abrupt event that endangers cerebral perfusion, either carotid clamping or hemodynamic troubles or displacement of the shunt. SEPs need about 1 min to build up an average response, and this restricts their use to situations where at least a little time is available to the surgeon for decision making. The best indication for the use of SEPs appears to be the question of to shunt or not to shunt, especially in situations when carotid occlusion induces ambiguous EEG deterioration. In these cases SEP provided the most helpful information. The rate of shunting has been decreasing since we used intraoperative SEP, without increasing the morbidity. The EEG however must be continuously monitored since it is common experience that not only the time of carotid occlusion affects the risk of brain ischemia: acute reductions of heart rate and arterial blood pressure may be relevant causes of stroke throughout the operation, and are more promptly identified by observation of EEG changes. Moreover, patients receiving temporary shunt are at the highest risk of brain ischemia; in these patients EEG can provide an early warning whenever something goes wrong while the shunt is inserted.

In conclusion, we think that double brain monitoring with EEG and SEP provides the best results by enhancing the advantages and reducing the pitfalls of either single technique. A sharpening of the intraoperative process of decision making in such high-risk surgery increases the safety of the procedure, not only when alarming information is forwarded, but also when a no-haste situation is promoted which helps the surgeon to work at his best.

References

1. Astrup J, Symon L, Branston NM et al. (1977) Cortical evoked potential and extracellular K+ and H+ at critical levels of brain ischemia. Stroke 8: 51–57
2. Astrup J, Symon L, Siesjo BK (1981) Threshold in cerebral ischemia – the ischemic penumbra. Editorial. Stroke 12: 723–725
3. Branston NM, Symon L, Crockard HA (1976) Recovery of the cortical evoked response following temporary middle cerebral artery occlusion in baboons: Relation to local blood flow and PO2. Stroke 7: 151–157
4. Chiappa KH, Burke SR, Young R (1979) Results of electroencephalographic monitoring during 367 carotid endarterectomies. Use of a dedicated minicomputer. Stroke 10: 1381–388
5. Cho I, Smullens SN, Streletz LJ, Fariello RG (1986) The value of intraoperative EEG monitoring during carotid endarterectomy. Ann Neurol 20: 508–512
6. Fava E, Bortolani E, Ducati A, Schieppati M (1992) Role of SEP in identifying patients requiring temporary shunt during carotid endarterectomy. Electroenceph Clin Neurophysiol 84: 426–432
7. Jacobs LA, Brinkman SD, Morrell LM, Shirley JG, Ganji S (1983) Long-latency somatosensory evoked potentials during carotid endarterectomy. Am Surg 49: 338–344
8. Jasper HH (1958) The ten-twenty electrode system of the International Federation. Electroenceph Clin Neurophysiol 10: 371–375
9. Jones TH, Morawetz RB, Crowell RM, Marcoux FW, Fitzgibbon SJ, De Girolami, U, Ojemann RG (1981) Thresholds of focal cerebral ischemia in awake monkeys. J Neurosurg 54: 773–782
10. McFarland HR, Pinkerton Jr JA, Frye D (1988) Continuous electroencephalographic monitoring during carotid endarterectomy. J Cardiovasc Surg 29: 12–18
11. McPherson RW, Johnson RM, Graf M (1983) Intraoperative neurological monitoring during carotid endarterectomy: electroencephalogram versus somatosensory evoked potentials. Anesthesiology 59: 368–373
12. Markand ON, Dilley RS, Moorthy SS, Warren C (1984) Monitoring of somatosensory evoked responses during carotid endarterectomy. Arch Neurol 41: 375–378
13. Prior PF (1985) EEG monitoring and evoked potentials in brain ischaemia. Br J Aaesth 57: 63–81
14. Russ W, Fraedrich G, Hehrlein FW, Hempelmann G (1985) Intraoperative somatosensory evoked potentials as a prognostic factor of neurologic state after carotid endarerectomy. Thorac Cardiovasc Surg 33: 392–396
15. Sundt TM, Sharbrough FW, Marsh WR, Ebersold MJ, Piepgras DG, Messick JM (1986) The risk-benefit ratio of intraoperative shunting during carotid endarterectomy. Relevancy to operative and postoperative results and complications. Ann Surg 203: 196–204
16. Trojaborg W, Boysen G (1973) Relation between EEG, regional cerebral blood flow and internal carotid artery pressure during carotid endarterectomy. Electroenceph Clin Neurophysiol 34: 61–69

Author's address:
E. Fava, MD
Istituto di Neurochirurgia
Università di Milano, Pad. Beretta Ovest
Via Francesco Sforza 35
20122 Milano, Italy

Transcranial Doppler sonography and internal carotid back pressure during carotid surgery: value, limits and results in comparison to somatosensory evoked potentials

M. Dinkel, H. Langer, P. Huber, H. Schweiger, W. Lang

Department of Anesthesiology and Division of Vascular Surgery, University of Erlangen-Nuremberg, Germany

In the preoperative period of carotid reconstructive surgery neither the neurological history nor angiographic examination enable us to identify patients at risk of ischemia due to insufficient collateral perfusion. Theoretically, this should be achievable by means of transcranial Doppler sonography (TCD) if there is evidence of impaired cerebrovascular reactivity, i.e., limited or no rise of blood flow velocity in the middle cerebral artery during carbon dioxide testing. But in their series of 93 procedures, Thiel and co-workers had to establish that 12 out of 13 patients with critical hypoperfusion and pathological somatosensory evoked potentials (SEP) during surgery showed preoperatively normal carbon dioxide reactivity, which would imply intact collateral perfusion. On the other hand, some 11 out of 80 patients with obvious patent collateral vessels and normal SEP response revealed pathological cerebrovascular reactivity (12).

Neuromonitoring: basic considerations

These observations underline the fact that, at the moment, impending intraoperative ischemia due to poor intracerebral collateral circulation cannot be identified preoperatively. On the other hand, the selective use of a temporary shunt and induced hypertension in patients with insufficient intracranial collateral blood flow is a rational strategy to avoid neurological complications during carotid surgery. This approach offers the opportunity to avoid the increased risk from categorical omission (i.e. cerebral ischemia) a well as the risks from general application of these measures (i.e. embolization with shunt placement, myocardial infarction due to induced hypertension and a false sense of safety if there is no intraoperative proof of effectivity). To put this strategy into clinical practice we need an intraoperative monitor, that identifies with a high sensitivity and specificity all patients with critical clamp-related ischemia. Furthermore, in order to be suitable for clinical routine application, a potential monitoring technique has to fulfill essential practical requirements (Table 4).

Somatosensory evoked potentials

One technique that meets nearly all requirements of an ideal monitor is the use of somatosensory evoked potentials (SEP) elicited by median nerve stimulation. This method is easy to perform with a low rate of failure (1–2 %) and is absolutely reliable as we could prove in a prospective study of 924 carotid operations (5). A loss of the cortical SEP response above the ipsilateral hemisphere after cross-clamping is a safe index of critical cerebral hypoperfusion (Fig. 1). In our experience this event occurs in only about 7 % of all procedures. Over 70 % of the patients not receiving a temporary shunt in this situation showed a transitory or permanent neurological deficit. Irreversible neurological dysfunction could, however, be prevented in all cases if a shunt was used that provided sufficient blood flow which could immediately be verified by recovering SEP amplitudes (Fig. 1) (5).

The high sensitivity and specificitiy of SEP monitoring in detecting clinically relevant clamp related ischemia is confirmed in various studies (2, 6, 7, 10, 12). Thus, SEP monitoring not only indicates the necessity of shunt placement reliably, but can also be taken as the gold standard in evaluating the significance of other cerebral monitoring techniques.

Transcranial doppler sonography

In this respect, the comparison with TCD in our own study showed good correlation between SEP findings and the blood flow velocity in the ipsilateral middle cerebral artery (v-mean MCA). Of 102 patients in whom we were able to perform simultaneous monitoring of SEP and TCD, only those five patients who also had a complete disappearance of

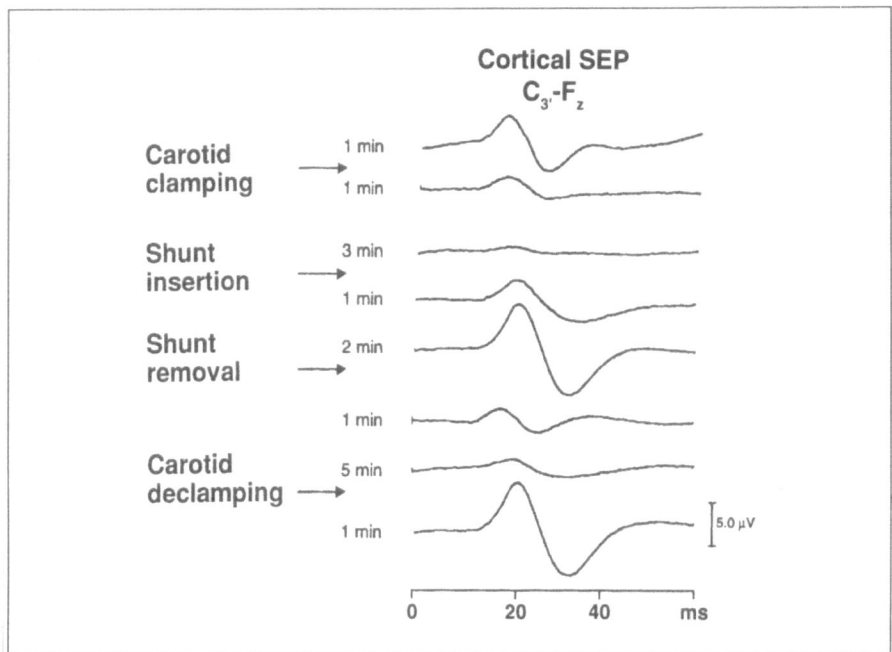

Fig. 1. Typical SEP recording during carotid surgery

the Doppler signal showed SEP loss (Table 1) (4). However, this unambiguous result is put into perspective by Thiel's findings. In some three patients with pathological SEP response after cross-clamping he could not find a critical reduction in middle cerebral artery blood flow velocity. On the other hand, he observed critical changes in TCD in 10 patients, two of whom even showed a complete loss of the signal, without evidence of pathological SEP changes or neurological deficits (12).

It is therefore obviously impossible to make safe predictions about the actual blood flow to functionally relevant areas from measuring blood flow velocity in basal cerebral arteries. Hence it is not surprising that the sufficiency of collateral perfusion cannot be determined reliably by TCD and that various studies produced dissimilar results when the question of the critical value of v-mean indicating cerebral ischemia was investigated (8, 9, 11, 12).

The main disadvantage of TCD, however, is a high rate of primary failure which was about 33 % in our own study (Table 2) (4). In another 10 % of cases we observed secondary dislocation of the ultrasound probe contributing to the fact that we could not use TCD to monitor cerebral blood flow during cross-clamping in altogether 43 % of patients. The number of patients in whom the MCA could not be identified a priori was especially

Table 1. Somatosensory evoked response and TCD findings during carotid artery cross-clamping (n = 102)

v-mean MCA	Cortical SEP	
	complete loss	identifiable
0 cm/s	n = 5	n = 0
> 0 cm/s	n = 0	n = 97

Table 2. Primary failure of TCD in relation to various disruptive factors

	Number	TCD Failure
Sex		
female	n = 58	n = 30 (51.7 %)**
male	n = 123	n = 29 (29.6 %)
Age		
< 70 years	n = 87	n = 19 (21.8 %)***
> 70 years	n = 94	n = 40 (42.6 %)
Neurological History		
asymptomatic	n = 35	n = 13 (37.4 %)
TIA	n = 102	n = 31 (30.4 %)
stroke	n = 44	n = 15 (34.1 %)
Contralateral Carotid Artery		
not stenotic (< 70 %)	n = 134	n = 45 (33.6 %)
stenotic (> 70 %)	n = 44	n = 14 (31.8 %)
SEP-findings		
identifiable	n = 162	n = 48 (29.6 %)*
complete loss	n = 19	n = 11 (57.9 %)
Total	n = 181	n = 59 (32.6 %)

*p < 0.05   **p < 0.01   ***p < 0.001

high among women, old people and patients who experienced SEP loss during the proce-dure (Table 2). The observation that TCD can be used successfully in less than 50 % of patients with insufficient collateral circulation raises serious questions about its usefulness as a monitor of ischemia (4).

This also puts into question the fact that by means of TCD there is a chance to identify hyperperfusion states and cerebral embolism as further causes of perioperative strokes. However, clinical interpretation of such TCD findings is in itself difficult. After declamp-ing many patients show an overshooting increase in v-mean MCA that normalizes within a few minutes and usually has no clinical consequences. This reaction probably reflects the process of adaptation of cerebral autoregulation to an increased cerebral blood flow after removal of the carotid stenosis. Therefore only long lasting hyperperfusion states which should be prevented by rigorous control of blood pressure, can be considered as patholog-ical (4, 11).

Even high frequency noise signals, which are a typical index of cerebral embolism, were seen in almost all patients shortly after release of the cross-clamp. However, we never detected any concomitant neurological deficit. This has also been observed in other clini-cal investigations (1, 9). There are several problems with detecting embolism by means of TCD. First despite new technological developments and promising data, it is still difficult to reliably disclose artefacts and to characterize the type of embolism. The critical number of embolic events that disturbs neurological function is still unknown. Finally, the most critical period of embolization is probably not intra- but postoperative.

Internal carotid back pressure

In contrast to TCD there is no failure with measurement of internal carotid back pressure (ICBP) (Table 4). In a series of 380 operations we noticed that as an indication of com-promised cerebral perfusion all patients with a loss of cortical SEP have ICBP levels that are only half of those obtained from patients with identifiable SEP, and we never could see pathological SEP findings if ICBP was in excess of 50 mmHg. However, about 50 % of all patients showed a critical ICBP below 50 mmHg without evidence of SEP alterations or neurological deficits indicating that ICBP is no reliable marker of cerebral perfusion (Table 3) (3). This is due to the same limitation that is true for TCD monitoring. Both techniques do not allow a safe estimation of the actual blood flow to brain areas prone to ischemia by measuring hemodynamic parameters at the skull base.

Table 3. Internal carotid back pressure compared to SEP findings after carotid cross-clamping (n = 380)

ICBP	Cortical SEP	
	complete loss	identifiable
≤ 50 mmHg	n = 40	n = 201
> 50 mmHg	n = 0	n = 139
Mean	19 mmHg	47 mmHg*
Range	10–41 mmHg	16–110 mmHg

*p < 0.001

Table 4. Cerebral monitors during carotid artery surgery

Requirements	SEP	TCD	CSP	EEG	SjO$_2$	rSO$_2$
Easy application	+	–	+	O	O	+
Low rate of failure	O	–	+	–	O	+
Continuous monitoring	+	+	–	+	+	+
Ease of interpretation	+	+	+	–	+	+
Unimpeded procedure	+	–	O	O	O	+
No side-effects	+	+	+	+	+	+
Affordable costs	+	+	+	+	–	O
High sensitivity	+	O	+	O	–	O
High specificity	+	O	–	O	–	–

Conclusions

Bearing all this in mind, it emerges that there are clear limitations to a profitable use of TCD and CSP measurement during carotid artery surgery. Both methods have only limited sensitivity and specifity with regard to critical cerebral ischemia. SEP monitoring, however, fits the essential requirements of a suitable neuromonitor. In this respect SEP is superior not only to TCD and ICBP but also to EEG, jugular bulb oximetry (SjO$_2$) and transcranial oximetry (rSO$_2$) (Table 4).

The high sensitivity reliably prevents ischemic neurological deficits. Sufficient shunt function is immediately indicated by recovering potentials. The high specificity of SEP minimizes risks of unnecessary shunt placement. As long as the cortical response can be evoked, there is no need for induced hypertension and cerebral integrity is not put at risk. This facilitates protection of heart and brain. SEP monitoring enables the surgeon to perform technically perfect surgery without undue haste. This provides further improvement of long-term results after carotis operations. And finally, the underlying mechanisms of neurological deficits are detected. A postoperative neurological deficit without intraoperative SEP loss points towards a source of embolism, meaning that there is a clear indication for surgical reexploration without further delay. These advantages contribute to a comparatively low rate of perioperative strokes (1.3 %) in our own group of patients. Thus SEP recording can be recommended as a routine monitor in carotid surgery.

References

1. Ackerstaff RGA, Jansen C, Moll FL, Vermeulen FEE, Hamerlijnck RPHM, Mauser HW (1995) The significance of microemboli detection by means of transcranial Doppler ultrasonography monitoring in carotid endarterectomy. J Vasc Surg 6: 963–969
2. Amantini A, Bartelli M, de Scisciolo G, Lombardi M, Macucci M, Rossi R, Pratesi C, Pinto F (1992) Monitoring of somatosensory evoked potentials during carotid endarterectomy. J Neurol 239: 241–247
3. Dinkel M, Schweiger H, Goerlitz P (1992) Monitoring during Carotid Surgery: Somatosensory Evoked Potentials vs. Carotid Stump Pressure. J Neurosurg Anesthesiol 4: 167–175
4. Dinkel M, Langer H, Loerler H, Rügheimer E, Schweiger H (1994) Neuromonitoring in der Karotischirurgie: Möglichkeiten und Grenzen der transkraniellen Doppler-Sonographie. VASA 23, 337–344

5. Dinkel M (1995) Funktionelles, hämodynamisches und metabolisches Neuromonitoring in der Karotis-chirurgie. Abbott, Wiesbaden
6. Fava E, Bortolani E, Ducati A, Schieppati M (1992) Role of SEP in identifying patients requiring temporary shunt during carotid endarterectomy. Electroenceph Clin Neurophysiol 84: 426–432
7. Gigli GL, Caramia M, Marciani MG, Zarola F, Lavaroni F, Rossini PM (1987) Monitoring of subcortical and cortical somatosensory evoked potentials during carotid endarterectomy: comparison with stump pressure levels. Electroenceph Clin Neurophysiol 68: 424–432
8. Halsey JH, McDowell HA, Gelmon S, Morawetz RB (1989) Blood velocity in the middle cerebral artery and regional cerebral blood flow during carotid endarterectomy. Stroke 20: 53–58
9. Jansen C, Vriens EM, Eikelboom BC, Vermeulen FEE, van Gijn J, Ackerstaff RGA (1993) Carotid Endarterectomy with Transcranial Doppler and Electroencephalographic Monitoring. Stroke 24: 665–669
10. Russ W, Fraedrich G, Hehrlein FW, Hemplemann G (1985) Intraoperative Somatosensory Evoked Potentials as a Prognostic Factor of Neurologic State after Carotid Endarterectomy. Thorac Cardiovasc Surgeon 33: 392–396
11. Spencer MP, Thomas GI, Moehring MA (1992) Relation Between Middle Cerebral Artery Blood Flow Velocity and Stump Pressure During Carotid Endarterectomy. Stroke 23: 1439–1445
12. Thiel A, Zickmann B, Stertmann WA, Wyderka T, Hempelmann G (1995) Cerebrovascular Carbon Dioxide Reactivity in Carotid Artery Disease. Anesthesiology 82: 655–661

Author's address:
Priv. Doz. Dr. med. M. Dinkel
Department of Anesthesiology
Friedrich Alexander University of Erlangen Nuremberg
Krankenhausstraße 12
91054 Erlangen, Germany

Use of EEG and TCD for assessment of brain function during operations on carotid artery

R. G. A. Ackerstaff[1], F. L. Moll[2]

Departments of Clinical Neurophysiology[1] and Vascular Surgery[2], St. Antonius Hospital, Nieuwegein (Utrecht), The Netherlands

Introduction

Since the first carotid artery reconstruction for transient ischaemic attack by Eastcott, Pickering, and Rob (1) in 1954, and the first successful carotid endarterectomy by DeBakey (2) in 1953, carotid endarterectomy has been commonly performed for prevention or relief of symptoms related to transient cerebral ischaemia. The ultimate goal of the operation is the prevention of stroke, and it is a diabolic paradox that the condition the operation is designed to prevent is also its most dreaded side-effect. Although the incidence of perioperative stroke is low in most currently reported series of carotid endarterectomies, no one has been able to completely eliminate this complication.

In the ongoing attempts to reduce morbidity and mortality in carotid surgery under general anaesthesia, a variety of intraoperative monitoring techniques have been developed to assess the need for increased cerebral protection. These techniques fall into two broad categories: 1) tests of vascular integrity as, for example, stump pressure measurements, Xenon regional cerebral blood flow (rCBF) studies, angioscopy, and transcranial Doppler (TCD) ultrasonography; and (2) tests of cerebral function as, for example, electroencephalography (EEG), EEG derivatives, and somatosensory evoked potential (SSEP) monitoring.

In this chapter we will describe the clinical relevancy of brain function monitoring during carotid endarterectomy by: (1) computerized EEG as a stand alone system, and (2) the supplementary value of TCD monitoring.

EEG expert system

In our institution we initially developed an EEG expert system for the automatic recognition of abnormal EEG activity during heart surgery and carotid endarterectomy (3, 4). For each patient a four channel strip chart is registered: fronto-parietal (F3/4-P3/4) and temporo-occipital (T3/4-O1/2) leads of each hemisphere are used. Additional to the strip chart registration, EEG signals are passed through a minicomputer. Besides the acquisition of the EEG, data concerning the blood pressure and anaesthesia used during surgery are recorded as well. Clinically relevant features are extracted from the EEG data and abnormal activity results in automatic warning and alarm signals, which are directly transmitted to the anaesthesiologist and the surgeon in the operating theatre. Trends in the patient data are presented in a graphical form (Fig. 1), and the instantaneously measured data,

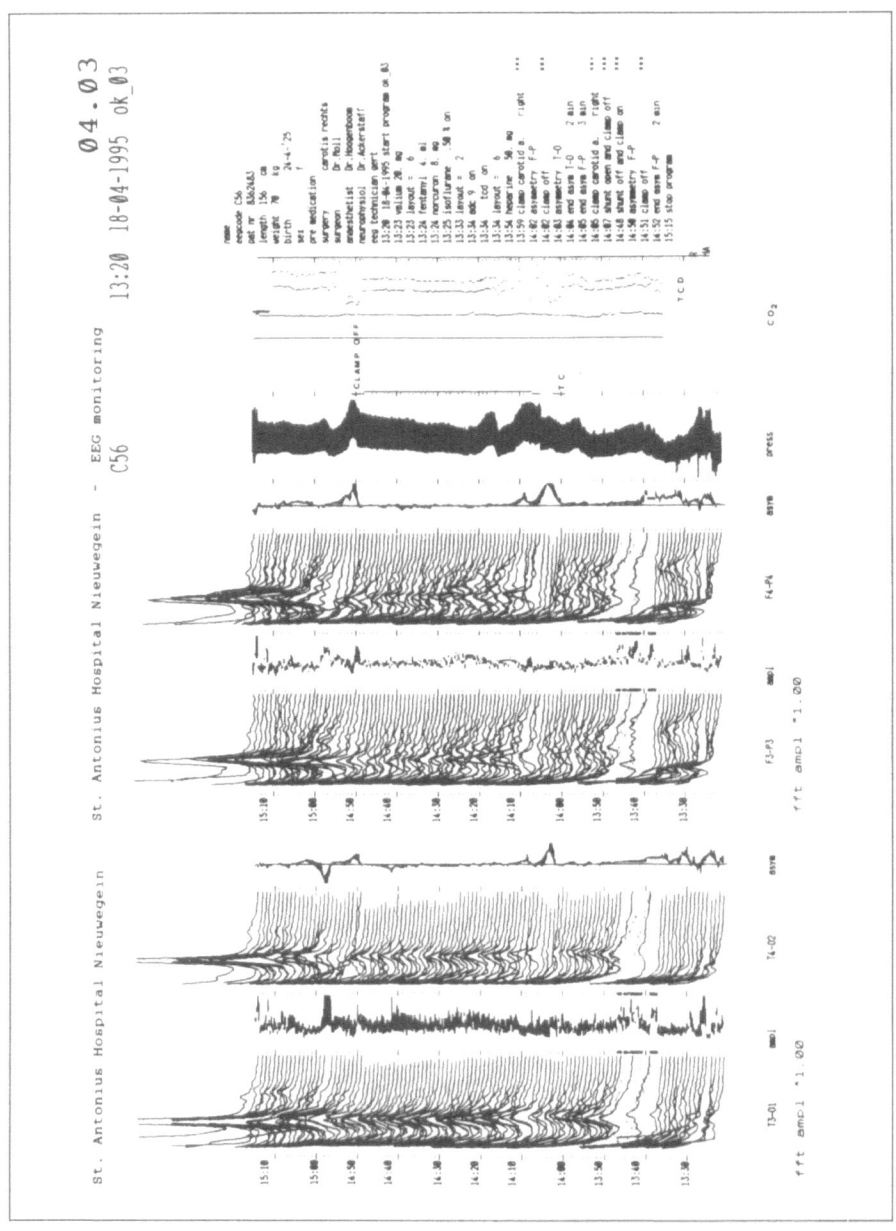

Fig. 1. A display of a multi-modal analysis of brain function during carotid endarterectomy with EEG as compressed spectral arrays of the temporo-occipital (T3-O1,T4-O2) and fronto-parietal (F3-P3,F4-P4) leads of both hemispheres, the asymmetry index (asym), blood pressure (press), end-tidal carbon dioxide tension (CO2), and peak and end diastolic MCA velocities (TCD). During test clamping (TC) of the right carotid artery, the EEG showed a severe asymmetry (AI > 20 %) and there was also a significant decrease of MCA velocities (80 %). Therefore, a shunt was used from 14.07 till 14.48. After the introduction of the shunt, the MCA velocities more or less restored to pre-clamp values. At cross-clamping for shunt removal, the EEG again showed a severe asymmetry, particularly in the fronto-parietal leads. During this operation the blood pressure was relatively unstable before and during the first 15 min of the arteriotomy, and after cross-clamp release (clamp off). During these periods, the TCD trend recording showed significant changes of MCA velocities parallel with changes of the blood pressure, indicating an autoregulatory dysfunction.

particularly the asymmetry between both hemispheres, are numerically displayed. The continuous blood pressure registration, which is directly related to the expected EEG data, makes it possible to maintain an adequate cerebral blood flow. The neurophysiologist has the opportunity of immediately comparing the graphically displayed data and the on line EEG which may be important in case of artifacts. In the development of this automatic EEG monitoring system we originally selected the period-amplitude analysis in which durations of zero-crossings of each hemisphere were converted to frequency. Later, this was replaced by fast Fourier transform of the EEG signal. In the latter format, the power of the EEG per unit of time has a strong relation with brain function and, therefore, gives a good indication of the functional status of the brain. The asymmetry of both the fronto-parietal and temporo-occipital leads is continuously calculated by using the following formula:

$$\frac{F75 \text{ left} - F75 \text{ right}}{F75 \text{ left} + F75 \text{ right}} \times 100\%$$

in which F75 left is the 75th percentile of the EEG power spectrum, measured during the last 15 s on the left side, and F75 right the one measured on the right side. Asymmetry between 15 % and 20 % is considered moderate, and asymmetry greater than 20 % severe.

In a retrospective analysis of 230 carotid endarterectomies, we evaluated the clinical relevancy of this EEG expert system (5). In this study, an indwelling shunt was selectively used on the basis of severe EEG asymmetry at cross-clamping. Attention was paid to the duration of the EEG asymmetry – transient or persistent – but also to the time interval between the onset of the EEG changes and the moment of cross-clamping. The purpose of this study was to analyse the importance of EEG changes with respect to intraoperative stroke in terms of predictive values, specificity, sensitivity, and diagnostic gain. The study demonstrated that a transient EEG asymmetry was never followed by a stroke. In 91 % of the cases with an EEG asymmetry at cross-clamping the asymmetry could be reversed by shunting. This underlines the haemodynamic aspect of transient EEG changes during carotid surgery and the benefit of shunting. On the other hand, persistent EEG asymmetry was strongly related to intraoperative major stroke (sensitivity 80 %, and specificity 99 %). Unfortunately, minor strokes were easily missed by our EEG expert system.

In cooperation with the University Hospital of Utrecht we reviewed perioperative strokes in 658 carotid endarterectomies (6) with the purpose of explaining the pathogenesis from the morphologic aspect of the infarct on cerebral computed tomograms (CT). In this series, there were 22 minor strokes (3.3 %) and 20 major strokes (3 %). Mortality was 0.8 %. Thirty-two percent of the CT-investigated strokes probably had a haemodynamic origin. Therefore, it was likely that the majority of intraoperative strokes (68 %) were of thromboembolic origin and primarily occurred during surgical manipulation of the carotid arteries.

To summarize, several conclusions can be drawn from these two retrospective studies:

1) With respect to the detection of intraoperative major stroke automatic EEG monitoring showed a good sensitivity and specificity. This was also expressed by the diagnostic gain of 47.8 %, indicating that the EEG contributes with an additional 47.8 % to the diagnosis of intraoperative major stroke. Therefore, it offers the possibility of taking the appropriate postoperative measures.

2) The selection of proper patients in the need of shunting on the basis of our EEG criteria was not perfect. After all, a considerable part of intraoperative strokes (32 %) probably had a haemodynamic origin.

3) Minor strokes and TIA's supposedly due to thromboembolic causes were only rarely detected by the EEG. Actually, this last conclusion was the main reason to add intra-operative TCD monitoring to our EEG expert system.

TCD monitoring

For the TCD registration a pulsed Doppler system with an improved monitoring trans-ducer with a 2 MHz emitting frequency (TC 2-64, TC 2000, or Pioneer TC 4040, EME, Überlingen, Germany) is used. Normally, the ipsilateral middle cerebral artery (MCA) is insonated through the transtemporal window and the sample volume is located at a depth of 45 to 55 mm. The probe is held in position using a plastic probe holder and elasticated head band protected by a detachable metal head guard which prevents dislodgement (Fig. 2). The audio Doppler signals are analyzed by a 128-point fast Fourier transform and it turned out to be important to make the Doppler signals audible in the operating theatre. Monitoring is continuous from commencement of anaesthesia till the end of the proce-dure. In addition, the Doppler signals are recorded onto digital audio tape for postopera-tive playback and analysis. Specially designed software (EME) allows individual time frames of the fast Fourier transform signals to be analysed. If embolic transients are recorded, this recording provides a measure of relative power amplitude in each successive

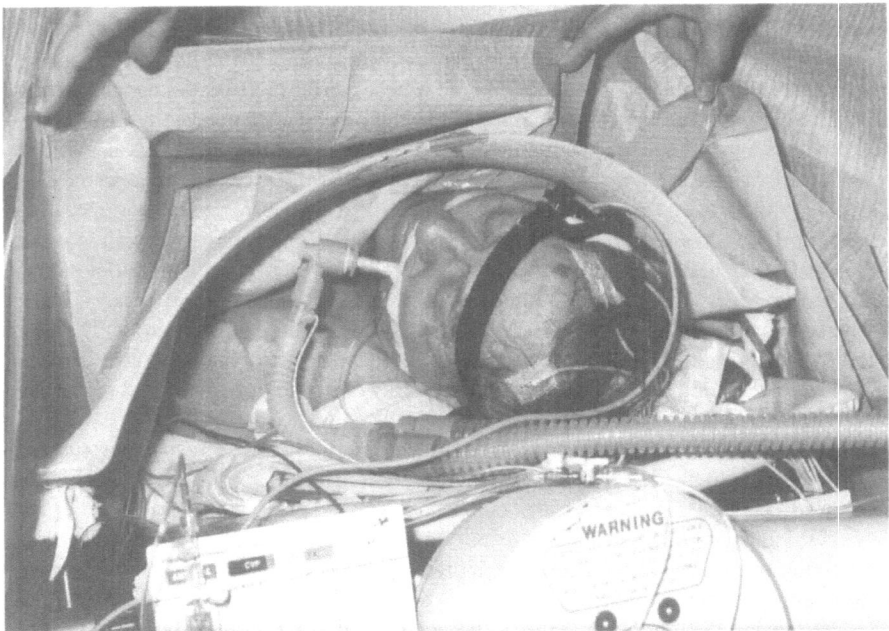

Fig. 2. The TCD transducer attached to the right side of the head of the patient with an elastic band and protected by a metal guard. Some of the EEG electrodes are also visible.

time frame. However, in all our studies the identification and counting of embolic transients are performed without the use of automatic emboli detection software, but rather through the continuous presence of a collaborator in the operating room for audio perception.

Haemodynamics of TCD monitoring

The MCA blood flow is recognized by its flow direction towards the probe, its high-pitched acoustic quality, and its attenuation during common carotid artery compression. Peak and mean blood flow velocities are measured continuously, as well as the pulsatility index. During carotid surgery, the most important moments of change of blood flow velocities occur at cross-clamping, cross-clamp release, and during the opening of a temporary shunt.

A few centres have described simultaneous brain function monitoring with EEG, rCBF, and TCD during carotid endarterectomy. In general, the relationship between rCBF measurements and MCA blood flow velocities is poor. Halsey (7, 8) reported that this relationship is dependent on the range of rCBF levels. The correlation was best at a rCBF level of less than 20 ml/100 g/min. Clamping in itself did not alter the relation, as it simply lowered both rCBF and MCA blood flow velocity. If rCBF was lowered to < 12 ml/100 g/min, the velocity waveform completely disappeared. The relatively poor correlation between the absolute values of MCA velocity and rCBF at cross-clamping is probably due to biological and methodological variability and can be partly eliminated by considering the relative decrease of MCA velocity. Using a 40 % decrease of MCA blood velocity at cross-clamping as a cut-off level, Jørgensen (9) correctly identified 89 % of the patients as having a rCBF above or below 20 ml/100 g/min. Similarly, using a 60 % decrease, 98 % of the patients were correctly diagnosed according to the appearance of EEG abnormalities.

Several important factors contribute to the spread of rCBF and MCA velocity measurements. Firstly, the relation between blood volume flow and velocity is not linear. Secondly, rCBF and MCA velocity are assessed in different regions of the brain. rCBF is calculated predominantly in the cortical convexity whereas MCA velocities are measured in the main stem of the MCA at the base of the brain. This also seems to be an explanation for the better correspondence of EEG changes with rCBF than with MCA velocities.

Since 1990, we have concomitantly used the above described computerised EEG expert system and TCD monitoring during carotid surgery (10, 11). In a series of 139 endarterectomies, the percentual decrease of peak and mean blood flow velocities at cross-clamping was compared with the EEG asymmetry calculated by the expert system. In this study, the only criterion used to select patients who are in need of a shunt was an EEG asymmetry index of more than 20 %. One-hundred-and-three patients demonstrated no EEG asymmetry at cross-clamping. In this group, the average reduction of mean blood flow velocities was 28.9 % (95 % confidence interval (CI): 24.9 % – 32.9 %). In the 19 patients with severe EEG asymmetry at cross-clamping, the average reduction of MCA velocities was 80.5 % (95 % CI: 70.3 % – 90.5 %). The difference between these two groups was statistically highly significant ($p < 10^{-6}$). ROC-analysis of the TCD data revealed that a 70 % decrease of MCA peak flow velocity resulted in a sensitivity of 84 % and a specificity of 96 %. For the reduction of the mean blood flow velocities the ROC curve parallelled the peak curve and showed an optimum cut-off level for a reduction of 65 % or more, corresponding with a sensitivity of 85 % and a specificity of 95 %. Using these cut-off values, there was only one case of false negative TCD data and in 6.5% of the cases the necessity of a shunt was overestimated.

From these studies, it gradually became clear that TCD monitoring provides additional and clinically relevant insight into haemodynamic changes of MCA blood flow velocities during cross-clamping. Although there was a significant correlation between EEG and TCD data during cross-clamping, not all TCD changes were reflected in the EEG expert system and vice versa. Some patients showed EEG changes without significant decrease of blood flow velocities, and other patients showed a dramatic reduction of blood flow velocities without EEG asymmetry. In our opinion, for selective shunting it is therefore important to take account of both monitoring methods at the same time. Because both modalities monitor different aspects of cerebral function, they are complementary with respect to the detection of cross-clamp ischaemia.

TCD monitoring and cerebral embolism

In the course of monitoring carotid endarterectomies with TCD ultrasonography it became apparent that during all stages of this operation signals identical to the qualities of embolic transients were noticed (10–15). It was clear that during arterial dissection before the arteriotomy these signals did not arise from gaseous emboli because it was not possible that air had been spontaneously entrained into the arteries. It was, therefore, concluded that these signals were caused by particulate emboli.

From our previous studies (10, 11) we concluded that the TCD technique has the unique potential to detect cerebral microemboli during carotid surgery. However, the occurrence of intraoperative microemboli without any clinical sequelae in the majority of our patients raised a fundamental question about the clinical relevancy of this phenomenon. If the effects of the detected microemboli in carotid endarterectomy cannot be demonstrated by means of neurological examination postoperatively, such effects might be shown by sensitive neuroimaging techniques. In the past 15 years CT has been the most common tool in the demonstration of cerebral lesions in clinically manifest or silent brain ischaemia. However, the introduction of magnetic resonance (MR) imaging has made it possible to detect in a very early phase even smaller ischaemic cerebral lesions, both in the cortex and the deep white matter (16–18). Moreover, new subcortical white matter hyperintensities on T2-weighted MR images have been described after therapeutic balloon occlusion of the internal carotid artery for unclippable giant aneurysms (19). Preoperative and postoperative MR scanning of the brain in patients who undergo carotid endarterectomy, therefore, seemed the most appropriate method for detection evidence of cerebral ischaemia caused by embolism.

To assess the impact of cerebral microembolism during carotid surgery on clinical outcome and brain architecture, 301 consecutive carotid endarterectomies were prospectively evaluated (20). All patients underwent neurologic examination before and after the operation. In a subgroup of 40 randomly selected endarterectomies, preoperative and postoperative cerebral MR imaging was made. The MR scans were made on a Philips Gyroscan T5 with a 0.5 Tesla superconducting magnet. After a T1-weighted spin echo scout view was obtained, axial T2-weighted spin echo images were made. The scans were made with a slice gap of 0.6 mm and a field view of 230 mm. We followed the same MR protocol during the preoperative and postoperative examinations and made every attempt to use an identical slice angulation. All MR scans were independently assessed by two radiologists. Microemboli were noticed in 69 % of all endarterectomies. This phenomenon varied from one single microembolus at the introduction of a needle for stump pressure measurement to a shower of microemboli of 5-min duration after release of the internal carotid artery cross-clamp. In 25 % of all endarterectomies microemboli occurred during dissection, which means they occurred before the arteries were opened. On the whole these phenomena were isolated microemboli related to surgical manipulation. In 5 % of these cases, more than 10 microemboli were noticed during dissection. Logistic regression analysis of preoperative and intraoperative risk factors showed that the phenomenon of more than 10 microemboli specifically during this stage of the operation had a statistically significant negative impact on clinical outcome. This phenomenon specifically resulted in intraoperative transient ischaemic deficits ($p < 0.002$). Of interest was that it also showed a significant correlation with postoperative ischaemic complications ($p < 0.02$). In the group of endarterectomies with preoperative and postoperative MR scanning of the brain, four (10 %) cases showed a new ischaemic lesion on the postoperative MR scan ipsilateral to the side of the operation. Three of these lesions were small, clinically silent, and deeply located hyperintensities on T2-weighted images. In this relatively small series of 40 patients, the phenomenon of more than 10 microemboli during the dissection phase was significantly correlated ($p < 0.005$) with the appearance of a new lesion on the postoperative MR scan. In this study, a shunt was used in 25 % (n = 76) of the operations. In 43 % of these shunted cases the use of a shunt resulted in the appearance of microemboli that were always less than 10. These shunt-related microemboli were significantly correlated with intraoperative ischaemic complications ($p < 0.007$). Finally, in 43 % of the operations microemboli were noticed at or after clamp release at the end of the arteriotomy. This phenomenon did not show a statistically significant relationship with perioperative complications.

Complications in the early postoperative phase

At present, in our institution the vast majority of perioperative cerebral complications in carotid surgery occur during the recovery period after the operation. Possible postoperative complications are an increase of thromboembolic events and thrombotic occlusion of the internal carotid artery. Neurologic events will appear only in cases with major cerebral embolization or if collateral perfusion is insufficient. If the TCD monitoring is extended into the postoperative period, both conditions can probably be determined (14, 21, 22). In particular, the study of Gaunt and co-workers (14) has highlighted the role of TCD in providing an early warning of incipient thrombosis in the immediate postoperative phase. However, experience with continuous TCD monitoring during the first hours after carotid surgery is limited and so far the conclusions are contradictory.

In addition, some neurologic complications after carotid endarterectomy occur in patients who were well after surgery for several days. Particularly the correction of high grade carotid artery stenosis in patients with severe multivessel disease and poor cerebral collateralization may be followed by ipsilateral headache, seizures, and in the worst case, intracerebral haemorrhage (ICH). These symptoms have been termed the postendarterectomy hyperperfusion syndrome. The neurological findings are attributed to abrupt increases in perfusion and loss of autoregulation due to chronic preoperative hypoperfusion contribute to the pathogenesis. With a decreasing perfusion pressure secondary to severe carotid artery stenosis and poor collaterals, the cerebral arterioles become maximally dilated and may lose their ability to constrict after normal perfusion pressure is restored. Autoregulatory failure and cerebral hyperperfusion occur for some time after carotid surgery, but as measurements by rCBF and TCD studies with hypercapnia and vasodilatation (CO_2 or Diamox) indicate, they eventually normalize during the first postoperative days (23, 24). Probably, the hyperperfusion syndrome after carotid surgery is more common than is now recognized (25). Jørgensen (24) showed that 18 % of her patients developed postendarterectomy hyperperfusion. In these patients, ipsilateral MCA blood flow velocity was blood pressure dependent. Moreover, she found an immediate cessation of symptoms with reduction of arterial pressure even in normotensive patients. In a study of 233 carotid endarterectomies, we compared the increase of MCA blood flow velocity at release of the internal carotid artery cross-clamp with the intraoperative preclamp value (26). Five patients (2.2 %) developed an ICH postoperatively. In this study, both the ICH group and the non-ICH group showed an increase of the ipsilateral MCA flow velocity on cross-clamp release. However, this increase was significantly higher ($p < 10^{-5}$) in the ICH group. Using simultaneously a 175 % increase of the peak flow velocity and a 100 % increase of the pulsatility index as cut-off values, the sensitivity, specificity, positive and negative predictive values, and the diagnostic gain with respect to the development of an ICH were respectively: 80 %, 100 %, 100 %, 99 %, and 98 %. Thus, using intraoperative TCD monitoring we could reliably identify patients at risk for ICH based on intraoperative factors occurring before the clinical symptoms. In our opinion, daily postoperative TCD examination should be performed in patients who demonstrate signs and symptoms of hyperperfusion. In these cases, careful postoperative management of hypertension is indicated.

Conclusion

The two retrospective studies on the reliability of our EEG expert system during carotid endarterectomy and on the pathogenesis of intraoperative infarcts (5, 6) showed that this system is not particular appropriate for the detection of minor stroke and TIA due to embolism related to surgical technique. However, we have to underline that this computerized system has a restricted spatial resolution. Instead of a complete 16-channel EEG, it only processes EEG data from two fronto-parietal and temporo-occipital leads. As yet, no data is available with respect to a minimum of EEG leads that is necessary for an accurate monitoring of brain function during carotid surgery.

The advantages of intraoperative TCD monitoring, such as its sensitivity for recording blood flow velocities and microembolism in real-time, are convincing. Because of its high temporal resolution it provides additional information about cerebral circulation, especially during cross-clamping and clamp release. Moreover, it may immediately detect shunt malfunction due to kinking or thrombosis and allow for correction before irreversible ischaemic damage has occurred. If made audible in the operating room, it also provides unique information to the surgeon concerning cerebral microembolization. Microemboli cause short transients in the Doppler spectral waveform that have characteristic acoustic properties and sound like bleeps, whistles, or clicks. Histologic examination of carotid specimens identified that ulcerated plaques with attached thrombus were significantly associated with TCD detected embolization during carotid artery dissection (27). In this respect, it is important to emphasize that in our studies most of the patients with multiple microemboli during the dissection phase showed only transient cerebral deficits or small, clinically silent lesions on MR imaging after the operation. In other words, the exact impact of cerebral microemboli on brain function and architecture is not yet completely understood, but particularly during dissection the embolic signals can warn the surgeon in time if manipulation of the carotid arteries causes embolism. Accordingly, the surgeon can try to adapt his or her technique to prevent a more serious outcome. For example, one solution is to stop the dissection, cross-clamp early and complete, possibly after insertion of an indwelling shunt, the dissection. It is not only our experience that surgeons can be guided by the "embolic signals" (15, 27, 28). Direct acoustic feedback to the surgeon can contribute to: 1) a more careful dissection of the artery, 2) a more scrupulous placing of the shunt, and 3) a more meticulous attention to backbleeding and flushing. When despite all these precautions a serious event happens, the best medical treatment and imaging of the carotid system (27) can be started without any delay. Since the introduction of TCD monitoring in our institution, the perioperative stroke rate declined from 4.8 % to 1 %.

Finally, TCD monitoring provides clinically relevant and useful information about potential postoperative complications, as for example postendarterectomy hyperperfusion, thrombosis, and occlusion of the internal carotid artery.

References

1. Eastcott HHG, Pickering GW, Rob CG (1954) Reconstruction of internal carotid artery in a patient with intermittent attacks of hemiplegia. Lancet, 994–996
2. DeBakey ME (1975) Successful carotid endarterectomy for cerebrovascular insufficiency: nineteen-year follow up. JAMA, 233, 1083–1085
3. Pronk RAF, Simons AJR (1982) Automatic recognition of abnormal EEG activity during open heart and carotid surgery. In: Kyoto Symposia (EEG suppl. no 36), ed. PA Buser, WA Cobb and T Okuma, Elsevier Biomedical Press, Amsterdam
4. Kniest EMM, Krul JMJ, Ackerstaff RGA (1989) Intra-operative EEG monitoring and stroke detection during carotid endarterectomy. Journal Electrophysiological Technology, 15, 21–26
5. Krul JMJ, Ackerstaff RGA, Eikelboom BC, Vermeulen FEE (1989) Stroke-related EEG changes during carotid surgery. European Journal Vascular Surgery, 3, 423–428
6. Krul JMJ, Gijn J van, Ackerstaff RGA, Eikelboom BC, Theodorides T, Vermeulen FEE (1989) Site and pathogenesis of infracts associated with carotid endarterectomy. Stroke, 20, 324–328
7. Halsey JH, McDowell HA, Gelman S (1986) Transcranial Doppler and rCBF compared in carotid endarterectomy. Stroke, 17, 1206–1208
8. Halsey JH, McDowell HA, Gelman S, Morawitz RB (1989) Blood velocity in the middle cerebral artery and regional cerebral blood flow during carotid endarterectomy. Stroke, 20, 53–58
9. Jørgensen LG, Schroeder TV (1992) Transcranial Doppler for detection of cerebral ischaemia during carotid endarterectomy. European Journal of Vascular Surgery, 6, 142–147
10. Jansen C, Vriens EM, Eikelboom BC, Vermeulen FEE, Gijn J van, Ackerstaff RGA (1993) Carotid endarterectomy with transcranial Doppler and electroencephalographic monitoring. A prospective study in 130 operations. Stroke, 24, 665–669
11. Jansen C, Moll FL, Vermeulen FEE, Haelst JMPI van, Ackerstaff RGA (1993) Continuous transcranial Doppler ultrasonography and electroencephalography during carotid endarterectomy: A multimodal monitoring system to detect introperative ischaemia. Annals of Vascular Surgery, 7, 95–101
12. Padayachee TS, Gosling RG, Bishop CC, Burnand K, Browse NL (1986) Monitoring middle cerebral artery blood velocity during carotid endarterectomy. British Journal of Surgery, 73, 98–100
13. Spencer MP, Thomas GI, Nicholls SC, Sauvage LR (1990) Detection of middle cerebral artery emboli during carotid endarterectomy using transcranial Doppler ultrasonography. Stroke, 21, 415–423
14. Gaunt ME, Martin PJ, Smith JL, Rimmer T, Cherryman G, Ratliff DA, Bell PRF, Naylor AR (1994) Clinical relevance of intraoperative embolization detected by transcranial Doppler ultrasonography during carotid endarterectomy: a prospective study of 100 patients. British Journal of Surgery, 81, 1435–1439

15. Ackerstaff RGA, Jansen C, Moll FL, Vermeulen FEE, Hamerlijnck RPHM, Mauser HW (1995) The significance of microemboli detection by means of transcranial Doppler ultrasonography monitoring in carotid endarterectomy. Journal of Vascular Surgery, 21, 963– 969

16. Buonanno FS, Pykett IL, Brady TJ, Vielma J, Burt CT, Goldman MR, Hinshaw WS, Pohost GM, Kistler JP (1983) Proton NMR imaging in experimental ischemic infarction. Stroke, 14, 178–184

17. Awad I, Modic M, Little JR, Furlan AJ, Weinstein M (1986) Focal parenchymal lesions in transient ischemic attacks: correlation of computed tomography and magnetic resonance imaging. Stroke, 17, 399–403

18. Kertesz A, Black SE, Nicholson L, Carr TH (1987) The sensitivity and specificity of MRI in stroke. Neurology, 37, 1580–1585

19. Awad IA, Masaryk T, Magdinec M (1993) Pathogenesis of subcortical hyperintense lesions on magnetic resonance imaging of the brain. Observations in patients undergoing controlled therapeutic internal carotid artery occlusion. Stroke, 24, 1339–1346

20. Jansen C, Ramos LMP, Heesewijk JPM van, Moll FL, Gijn J van, Ackerstaff RGA (1994) Impact of micro-embolism and haemodynamic changes in the brain during carotid endarterectomy. Stroke, 25, 992–997

21. Laman DM, Voorwinde A, Davies G, Duijn H van (1989) Intraoperative internal carotid artery restenosis detected by transcranial Doppler monitoring. British Journal of Surgery, 76, 1315–1316

22. Zuilen EV van, Moll FL, Vermeulen FEE, Mauser HW, Gijn J van, Ackerstaff RGA (1995) Detection of cerebral microemboli by means of trans-cranial Doppler monitoring before and after carotid endarterectomy. Stroke, 26, 210–213

23. Bishop CC, Butler L, Hunt T, Burnand KG, Browse NL (1987) Effect of carotid endarterectomy on cerebral blood flow and its response to hypercapnia. British Journal of Surgery, 74, 994–996

24. Jørgensen LG, Schroeder TV (1993) Defective cerebrovascular autoregulation after carotid endarterectomy. European Journal of Vascular Surgery, 7, 370–379

25. Breen JC, Caplan LR, DeWitt LD, Belkin M, Mackey WC, O'Donnell TP (1996) Brain edema after carotid surgery. Neurology, 46, 175–181

26. Jansen C, Sprengers AM, Moll FL, Vermeulen FEE, Hamerlijnck RPHM, Gijn J van, Ackerstaff RGA (1994) Prediction of intracerebral haemorrhage after carotid endarterectomy by clinical criteria and intra-operative transcranial Doppler monitoring: Results of 233 operations. European Journal of Vascular Surgery, 8, 220–225

27. Gaunt ME, Brown L, Hartshorne T, Bell PRF, Naylor AR (1996) Unstable carotid plaques: Preoperative identification and association with intraoperative embolisation detected by transcranial Doppler. European Journal of Vascular and Endovascular Surgery, 11, 78–82

28. Gaunt ME, Smith JL, Ratliff DA, Bell PRF, Naylor AR (1996) A comparison of quality control methods applied to carotid endarterectomy. European Journal of Vascular and Endovascular Surgery, 11, 4–11

Author's address:
R. G. A. Ackerstaff, MD, Ph D
St. Antonius Ziekenhuis
Dept. of Clinical Neurophysiology
Koekoekslaan 1
3435 CM Nieuwegein, The Netherlands

Intraoperative monitoring in carotid surgery: transcranial Doppler versus somatosensory evoked potential method

S. Ricke, K. Ktenidis, K. Heye, S. Horsch

Krankenhaus Porz am Rhein, Department of Vascular Surgery,
Academic Teaching Hospital of University of Cologne

Introduction

In the industrialised countries of the western world cerebrovascular insufficiency is the third most common disease affecting the general population following cardiac disease and cancer. Relevant statistics qualify cardiovascular disease as the leading cause of death in 40 % of cases. Of those affected, one-third die due to myocardial or cerebral infarction (6). The diagnosed new cases every year with disease of the supraaortic vessels increases exponentially with the patients' gain in age: roughly 300 cases per 100000 in the age group 55 to 64 years and 1440 cases in the age category 75 to 84 years. Above 85 years a prevalence of 2000 per 100000 has been documented (2, 5, 9). The expected stroke rate in the population therefore correspondingly rises with the currently increasing mean population age of western societies. Two-thirds of the patients who survive a stroke are handicapped by the incident, and 10 % of these require full-time care (12). Half of these patients survive another 5 years, and one-third of these require prolonged rehabilitation in specially equipped centres. The cost of caring for these patients in the United States is estimated to lie at 9 Million US $ per year. Roughly 75 % of the extracranial arterial lesions can be reconstructed in vascular surgical procedures in order to achieve an adequate cerebrovascular circulation. The cost for this type of treatment in the states was calculated to be 1.25 Million US $ compared to the above mentioned figures (8).

Based on the principle that the surgical procedure may not have more risk than the uninterrupted natural course of the disease, it is of particular importance to adequately monitor the intracerebral perfusion during the reconstruction period of the internal carotid artery in order to avoid perioperative complications.

Despite controversial discussions, carotid endarterectomy has become an established method in vascular surgery, demanding a careful indication, subtle technique and intraoperative monitoring of cerebral function and perfusion. The controversy is regarding intraluminal shunt insertion as well as early recognition of intraoperative complications, such as malperfusion of cerebral tissue leading to ischaemia, possible embolisation, shunt occlusion or dislocation of the shunt with consecutive postoperative neurological deficit. The foregoing has lead to a search since the 1960s to obtain reliable and objective methods of monitoring during carotid surgery.

Due to the lack of reliability and the immense technical and personnel display of stump-pressure measurement of the internal carotid artery and electroencephalography as monitoring devices during carotid surgery, transcranial Doppler ultrasound (TCD) and measurement of the somatosensory evoked potentials (SEP) were introduced. The SEP supplies more information on cerebral function, whereas the TCD provides valuable data about the intracerebral haemodynamic situation (1, 3, 4, 7, 11). In a prospective study we examined from January 1988 to December 1993 the reliability of SEP- and TCD methods for intraoperative monitoring during carotid endarterectomy. The aim was to determine the risk of cerebral ischaemia during the clamping period, the necessity of intraluminal shunt insertion and to register intraoperative complications such as embolisation or dysfunction of a shunt.

Materials and methods

From January 1988 to December 1993 we performed 714 carotid endarterectomies under general anaesthesia using SEP and TCD simultaneously for intraoperative monitoring on 653 patients. In our patient group we had 414 males and 239 females. The mean age was 67.3 years; 43 % of patients were asymptomatic, 9 % had suffered an asymptomatic infarction visible on CCT-scan, 39 % had a transient ischemic attack, 2 % had a prolonged reversible ischaemic neurological deficit (PRIND) and 7 % a fulminant stroke preoperatively. Routine preoperative diagnosis included duplex scanning, digital subtraction angiography of the supraaortic vessels and CCT. Furthermore the degree of stenosis was reassessed intraoperatively; 14 % of cases had a stenosis of < 75 % , 39 % a 75–90 % stenosis, 46 % a stenosis of > 90 % and 1 % a complete occlusion of the internal carotid artery.

Somatosensory evoked potentials were derived from the ipsilateral cortex after stimulation of the contralateral median nerve at the wrist for assessment of the N20/P25 amplitude. Electrodes were placed in the middle of the forehead, behind the ear and a distance of 4×2 cm away (parieto-occipital) from this point corresponding to the somatosensory cortical protection fields and according to the 10–20 International System.

Transcranial Doppler assessment permits noninvasive determination of the intracranial arterial flow velocity. Changes in flow velocity are expected to correspont to cerebral blood flow, provided the vessel diameter, flow profile and the angle between the ultrasound beam and the vessel remain relatively constant. There is, however, a wide range among patients, possibly related to physiological variations, as well as in the diameter of the intracranial vessels. However, for continuous and noninvasive monitoring during carotid surgery in specific patients, TCD provides instantaneous information on changes in flow velocity, primarily in the middle cerebral artery (MCA). TCD was performed transtemporally. The flow velocity was measured in the main branch of the middle cerebral artery through a temporal bone window. The first registration was documented just prior to surgical intervention. During the operation, TCD was measured immediately before and during the first clamping, after introduction of a necessary shunt and during the second clamping after shunt removal.

Results

During 714 carotid endarterectomies (653 patients) transcranial Doppler and measurement of somatosensory evoked potentials could be registrated simultaneously: 411 cases showed no significant reduction of flow velocity, 84 a reduction of ≤ 59 % and 78 a reduction ≤ 69 %. In summary an abnormal MCA flow reduction was noticed in 141 cases corresponding to a shunt rate of 20 % (Fig. 1).

Previously, according to other statistics and publications, we defined a reduction of MCA flow of > 50 % as pathological, but currently we have applied a definition of a flow reduction > 70 % as pathological. Of the 714 endarterectomies performed, a flow reduction of 50–69 % was documented in 162 cases. Only 5 cases developed a pathological SEP curve in this patient group. Of the 141 cases with a > 70 % reduction in flow velocity, 64.5 % has a corresponding pathological SEP curve (Fig. 2).

In our patient group with simultaneous TCD and SEP monitoring during carotid endarterectomy, 0.9 % suffered a stroke, 0.6 % a PRIND and 2.1 % a transient ischaemic attack. The mortality rate was 1.9 %. Combining the SEP and TCD monitoring the statistical analysis showed a sensitivity of 96 %, a specificity of 92 %, a positive predictive value of 64.5 % and a negative predictive value of 99.5 %.

Discussion

Due to the high rate of false positive TCD measurements the threshold value for pathological reduction of flow velocity of the MCA should be > 50 %. When increased to 70 % we noticed a simultaneously pathological SEP in 64.5 % of cases. This seems to justify correlating a decrease of flow velocity of > 70 % with an inadequate intracerebral collateralisation, demanding the use of an intraluminal shunt.

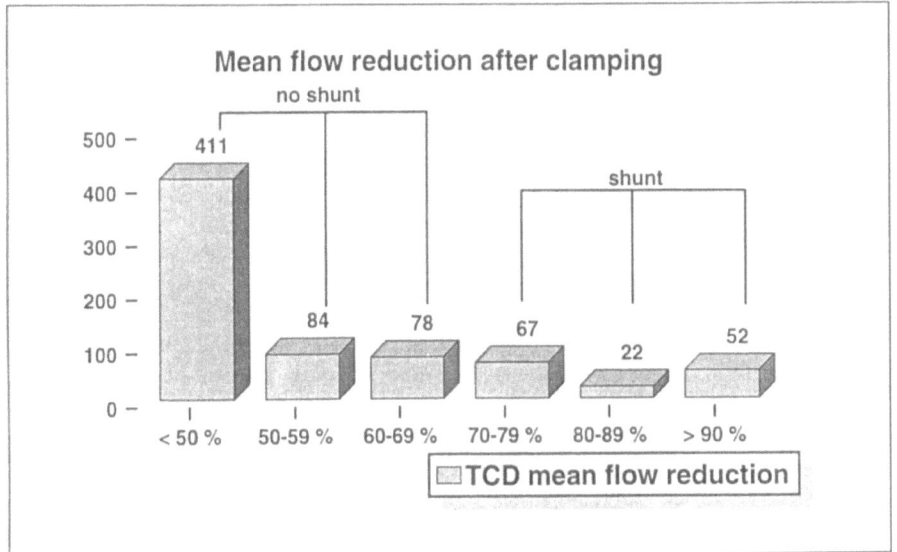

Fig. 1. Transcranial Doppler (TCD)

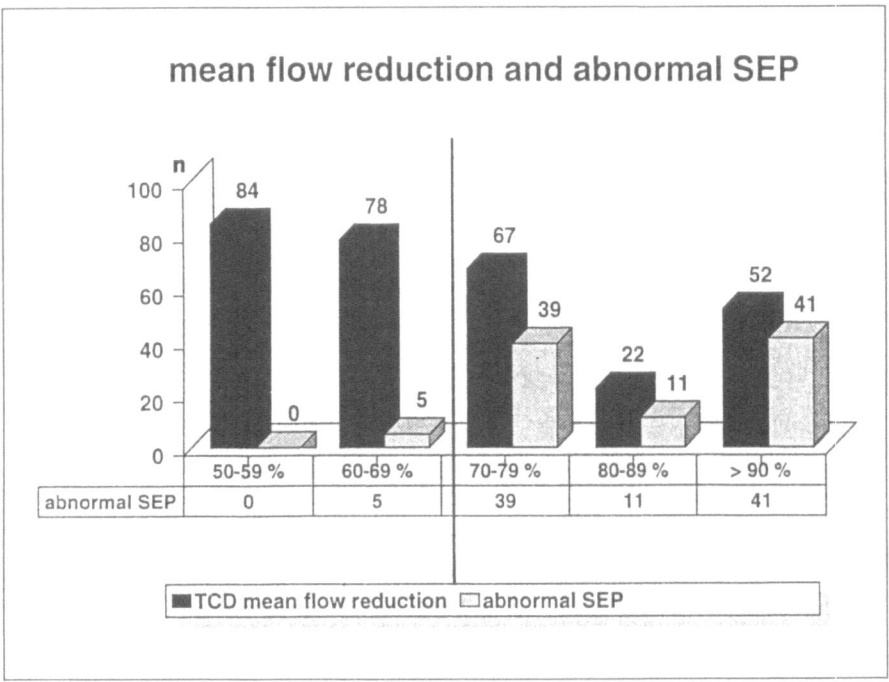

Fig. 2. TCD vs SEP monitoring

In our opinion the combined use of SEP and TCD as monitoring during the carotid endarterectomy delivers precise information about the effect of clamping on brain function and cerebral hemodynamics. The indication for an intraluminal shunt insertion during the surgical procedure should rely on the N20/P25 amplitude during the test clamping and a loss of SEP-amplitude of > 50 % during carotid artery clamping. TCD can also determine the necessity of a shunt by evaluating the clamping effect. A reduction of > 70 % of mean flow velocity demands the insertion of an intraluminal shunt to adequately protect the brain from ischemic damage. However TCD cannot recognize major complications during surgery such as distal embolisation and therefore should not be used alone in carotid surgery.

The aim of intraoperative monitoring is to reduce the incidence of neurological morbidity by identifying cerebral ischaemia and implementing measures to obviate ischaemia while it is still reversible. Embolic events and postoperative thrombosis may not be prevented by monitoring, but may be recognized before they manifest themselves clinically. Only hypoperfusion during occlusion may be identified and prevented by insertion of a temporary indwelling shunt.

Due to the lack of conclusive data, carotid surgeons tend to swear by one of three shunt policies: to insert a shunt routinely, to insert a shunt selectively or to never use a shunt. In our opinion selective shunting yields the lowest complication rate, provided a reliable monitoring technique, such as combined SEP and TCD assessment, is available.

References

1. Aaslid R, Markwalder TM, Nornes H (1982) Noninvasive transcranial Doppler ultrasound recording of flow velocity in the basal cerebral arteries. J Neurosurg 57: 769–774
2. Bonita R (1992) Epidemiology of stroke. In: Stroke octet from the Lancet. A review, pp 1–3
3. Burmeister W, Doerrler J, Maurer PC, Mix C (1987) Transcranielles Doppler Monitoring bei rekonstruktiven Eingriffen an der Carotisgabel. Angio 9: 231
4. De Vleeschauwer PH, Horsch S, Matamoros R (1988) Monitoring of somatosensory evoked potentials in carotid surgery: results, usefullness and limitations of the method. Ann Vasc Surg 2: 63
5. Garraway WM, Whisnant JP, Furian AJ (1979) The declining incidence of stroke. N Engl J Med 300: 449
6. Heberer G (1978) In: Heberer G (ed) Die Arteriosklerose als chirurgische Aufgabe. TM-Verlag, Bad Oeynhausen
7. Markand ON, Dilley RS, Moorthy SS, Warren C Jr (1984) Monitoring of somatosensory evoked responses during carotid endarterectomy. Arch Neurol 41: 375–378
8. Mayo Asymptomatic Carotid Endarterectomy Study Group (1989) Effectiveness of carotid endarterectomy for asymptomatic carotid stenosis: Design of a clinical trial. Mayo Clin Proc 64: 897
9. Mc Dowell FH, Caplan LR (1985) Cerebrovascular survey report for the National Institutes of Neurologic and Communicative Disorders and Stroke. National Institute of Health, Public Health Service, Bethesda, Md
10. Padayachee TS, Gosling DG, Lewis RR, Bishop CC, Browse NL (1987) Transcranial Doppler assessment of cerebral collateral during carotid endarterectomy. Br J Surg 74: 260–262
11. Schneider PA, Ringelstein B, Rossmann ME, Dilley RB, Sobel DF, Otis SM, Bernstein EF (1988) Importance of cerebral collateral pathways during carotid endarterectomy. Stroke 19: 1328
12. Wolf PA, Dawber TR, Thomas HE (1977) Epidemiology of stroke. In: Thompson RA, Green JR (eds) Advances in neurology. Raven Press, New York, pp 5–19

Author's address:
S. Ricke, M.D.
Krankenhaus Porz am Rhein
Department of Vascular Surgery,
Academic Teaching Hospital of University of Cologne
Urbacher Weg 19
51149 Cologne, Germany

Transcranial cerebral oxymetry versus jugular venous oxygen saturation

G. Grubhofer

Klinik für Anästhesie Wien, Austria

The benefit of carotid thrombendarterectomy in the treatment of carotid artery disease has been confirmed by major clinical trials (2, 7). In order to prevent ischemic brain damage during temporary occlusion of the carotid artery, the adequacy of collateral flow may be monitored by several means (6). This includes:
▶ brain function (EEG recording, SEPs)
▶ cerebral blood flow and perfusion (transcranial Doppler ultra-sonography)
▶ regional cerebral oxygenation (RSO2), jugular venous bulb oxygenation (Sjo2).

During carotid crossclamp, followed by cerebral hypoperfusion, all these measures will decrease. Usually, not all of these cerebral monitoring methods will be available in clinical practice. Nevertheless, if a good correlation between the measured values can be proven, one method can in part replace the others.

In contrast to arterial oxygenation, cerebral venous oxygenation (= jugular venous bulb oxygenation) (SjO2) reflects the adequacy and amount of global cerebral blood flow. The interrelationship between cerebral venous oxygenation and flow can be described by the following simplified formula:

$$SjO2 \sim \text{cerebral blood flow} / \text{cerebral oxygen consumption}$$

As cerebral oxygen consumption can be assumed to remain unchanged during anesthesia, SjO2 remains a direct measure of cerebral blood flow. The normal values of SjO2 range between 60 % and 75 %. Values below 50 % will be followed by mental disordering and slowing of electrical activity. SjO2 values can be obtained continuously by introducing a catheter (Opticath 4f, Oximetrix) retrogradely into the internal jugular vein.

Recently, a monitor was developed (Invos 3100, Somanetics) to measure regional cerebral oxygenation (RSO2) using the principle of near infrared spectroscopy. Measured values of RSO2 are reported to correlate closely with SjO2. The clinical importance and usefulness of both RSO2 and SjO2 is well proven in head injured patients (12). Thus, RSO2 and SjO2 are considered to have important applications also during carotid surgery (1, 4, 5).

However, before a new monitoring device can even be considered for clinical use, the accuracy, precision, sensitivity, specificity, cutoff point definition, and other essential characteristics have to be proven (10). Determining the accuracy of RSO2 is difficult as the obtained values cannot be directly calibrated with a "gold standard" reference parameter. At present, the most precise clinical reference parameter is the jugular venous bulb (SjO2) oxygen saturation (5, 8) used in most validation studies.

Tateishi (11) induced increases in cerebral blood flow by altering PaCO2, an intervention generally considered to alter only cerebral blood flow. The direction and magnitude in changes of RSO2 were similar to changes of SjO2 suggesting sufficient accuracy of both methods to estimate cerebral perfusion. During carotid surgery, Williams (13) found a good correlation between changes in RSO2 and flow velocities in the middle cerebral artery determined by transcranial Doppler sonography. In healthy volunteers also Pollard (8) observed a close correlation between RSO2 and estimated combined brain oxygenation (a value obtained from SjO2 and arterial oxygenation). The authors conclude that RSO2 is a simple noninvasive technique for continuously monitoring brain oxygenation.

In other studies, however, considerable doubts have been expressed concerning the accuracy of measured RSO2 values (10). Harris (3) did not observe a change in RSO2 during increases in middle cerebral artery flow-velocity. Thus the authors conclude that RSO2 reflects external carotid flow in the scalp and skull with minimal contribution from the internal carotid circulation.

Having a closer look into the principle of RSO2 measurements, this could be a serious limitation of this technique. The now available device (Invos 3100) measures cerebral oxygen saturation continously by spectroscopy of reflected near infrared light. The sensor consists of one light transmitter and two detectors. Near infrared light (wavelengths 650 and 1100 nm) penetrates tissues and will be reflected in a parabolic curve. One detector is designed to receive light predominately from superficial areas of the scalp, skull and the brain, while the more distant detector should receive light especially from deep brain areas. From both signals, a computer calculation estimates pure cerebral oxygenation.

"Pollution" of RSO2 values by extracranial tissue oxygenation is assumed but not proven to be eliminated by a source to detector separation distance of 30 and 40 mm, which is the currently available sensor type (13). To determine the relative contribution of extracranial tissue oxygenation on RSO2 values, we designed a study during carotid thrombendarterectomy, measuring blood oxygenation drawn from the facial vein (S-extO2) as well as the jugular venous bulb (SjO2). Blood from extracranial forehead areas drains substantially into the facial vein. Thus, the extent of extracranial contribution can be quantified by comparing blood oxygenation drawn from this vein with RSO2 values.

Using linear regression analyses, we found no dependency of RSO2 on S-extO2 ($p = 0.35$), but a significant dependency of RSO2 on SjO2 ($p = 0.007$). Thus we consider the influence of extracranial tissue oxygenation to be small on measured RSO2 values. Can we conclude from this that RSO2 is a useful monitor of cerebral oxygenation during carotid surgery? I think we cannot. To present, no clear critical value of RSO2 has been defined at which cerebral hypoxia and ischaemia is possible. Due to this problem, most investigators emphasize that not absolute values of RSO2 should used for cerebral monitoring, but changes in these values should give clinically relevant information (1, 13).

In our data, changes in RSO2 reflected global brain oxygenation (SjO2) inaccurately. RSO2 data were moderately sensitive only to decreases in SjO2. Increases in SjO2, on the other hand, led to unpredictable changes in RSO2. As for decreasing RSO2 values, the corresponding SjO2 data decreased in only 70 % of cases, SjO2 increased in the remaining 30 %. This indicates that RSO2 predictions regarding global brain oxygenation was wrong in 30 % of cases and would be misleading in clinical practice if used alone. There are two possibile explainations for these discrepancies in the accuracy of RSO2 data.

First, RSO2 and SjO2 measure two different aspects of cerebral oxygenation, which are related but not identical. Currently, RSO2 values indicate the oxygenation in mixed arterial, capillary and venous blood. Therefore, RSO2 changes can result from a change in arterial saturation, venous saturation, altered proportions of blood within the arterial, capillary and venous compartments or a combination of these. Cerebral blood volume distribution is usually 25 % arterial, 5 % capillary and 70 % venous (9). These proportions however are likely to vary in case of cerebrovascular disease, anesthesia and otherwise pathological conditions.

Second, RSO2 data only reflect the local condition of the frontal lobe. Changes in other brain areas will escape detection. In contrast, SjO2 provides information on global brain oxygenation. Any spotty, inhomogeneous distribution of blood and metabolic activity will therefore reduce the correlation between these two measurements.

In conclusion, our results show influence of extracranial tissue oxygenation on measured RSO2 values is insignificant during carotid thrombendarterectomy. The accuracy of RSO2 values to detect cerebral hypoxia, however, remains uncertain, as changes in global brain oxygenation are not always correctly identified.

Owing these limitations, it would be inappropriate to interpret RSO2 values alone as a reflection of cerebral oxygenation. Thus, the values obtained from Invos 3100 should be used only in conjunction with other techniques, to provide an early warning of inadequate cerebral flow during carotid thrombendarterectomy.

References

1. Duncan LA, Ruckley CV, Wildsmith JAW (1995) Cerebral oximetry: a useful monitor during carotid artery surgery. Anaesthesia 50: 1041–45
2. European carotid surgery trialists' collaborative group (1991) MRC European carotid surgery trial: interim results for symptomatic patients with severe (70–99 %) or with mild (0–29 %) carotid stenosis. Lancet 337: 1235–1243
3. Harris DNF, Bailey SM (1993) Near-infrared spectroscopy in adults. Does the Invos 3100 really measure intracerebral oxygenation? Anaesthesia 48: 694–696
4. Kirkpatrick PJ, Smielewski P, Whitfield PC, Czosnyka M, Menon D, Pickard JD (1995) An observational study of near-infrared spectroscopy during carotid endarterctomy. Journal of Neurosurgery 82: 756–763
5. Mc Cormick P, Stewart M, Goetting MG, Balakrishnan G (1991) Regional cerebrovascular oxygen saturation measured by optical spectroscopy in humans. Stroke 22: 596–602
6. Naylor AR, Bell PRF, Ruckley CV (1992) Monitoring and cerebral protection during carotid endarterectomy. British Journal of Surgery 79: 735–741
7. North American symptomatic carotid endarterecatomy trial collaborators (1991) Beneficial effect of carotid endarterctomy in symptomatic patients with high-grade carotid stenosis. New England Journal of Medicine 325: 445–453
8. Pollard V, Prough DS, Demelo AE, Deyo DJ, Uchida T, Stoddart HF (1996) Validation in volunteers of a near-infrared spectroscope for monitoring brain oxygenation in vivo. Anesthesia & Analgesia 82: 269–277
9. Portnoy HD, Chopp M (1994) Intracranial fluid dynamics. Interrelationship of CSF and vascular phenomena. 1983. Pediatric-Neurosurgery 20: 92–98
10. Prough DS, Pollard V (1995) Cerebral near-infrared spectroscopy: Ready for prime time? Critical Care Medicine 23: 1624–1626
11. Tateishi A, Maekawa T, Soejima Y, Sadamitsu D, Yamamoto M, Matsushita M, Nakashima K (1995) Qualitative comparison of carbon dioxide-induced change in cerebral near infrared spectroscopy versus jugular venous oxygen saturation in adults with acute brain desease. Critical Care Medicine 23: 1734–1738
12. Unterberg A, Rosenthal A, Schneider GH, Kiening K, Lanksch WR (1995) Validation of monitoring of cerebral oxygenation by near-infrared spectroscopy in comatose patients. In: Tsukobawa T, Marmarou A, Robertson C, Teasdale G (eds) Neurochemical Monitoring in the Intensive Care Unit. Tokyo: Springer
13. Williams IM, Picton A, Farrell A, Mead GE, Mortimer AJ, Mc Collum N (1994) Light reflective cerebral oximetry and jugular bulb venous oxygen saturation during carotid endarterectomy. British Journal of Surgery 81: 1291–1295

Author's address:
Dr. G. Grubhofer
AKH Wien
Klinik für Anästhesie & Allg. Intensivmedizin
Währinger Gürtel 18
1080 Wien, Austria

Transcranial cerebral oxymetry (TCO): a valid monitoring method during carotid surgery?

K. Ktenidis, K. Simons, S. Horsch

Department of General and Vascular Surgery, Krankenhaus Porz am Rhein, Academic Teach.-Hospital of the University of Cologne, Germany

Introduction

Present-day discussions amongst specialists show that carotid surgery has to stand up to constantly increasing demands. Apart from strict guidelines for surgical indications as well as involved surgical technique, the necessity of perioperative monitoring is increasingly stressed (5). The monitoring during carotid reconstructions is particularly demanded. The significance of this monitoring consists of evaluating of the clamping effect, determining the necessity of using a shunt, evaluating of the effectiveness of the shunt, timely recognition of intraoperative complications, and the insurance of operative quality.

We report about experiences using cerebral oxymetry as a monitoring method during carotid surgery. The aim of our study was to determine the reliability of this method, its sensitivity and specificity, as well as positive and negative predictive value. Another reason for this study was to determine the measure of the critical reduction of oxygen saturation in the brain measured transcranially.

Materials and methods

With the aid of a new developed infrared-spectroscopy (INVOS 3100, Somanetics), the transcranial oxygen saturation of cerebral blood is measured. A near infrared emitter and receiver is placed over the temporo-frontal brain on the scalp (Fig. 1). Briefly, infrared light of the region between 750-950 nm is transmitted sufficiently through the soft and hard tissues of the head to provide an adequate signal for spectrophotometric purposes. The signal from receiver #1 can be used to correct the signal from receiver #2 for superficial contamination. Using near-infrared spectroscopy, regional oxygen saturation (rSO2) of the brain with minimal extracerebral contamination can be monitored during carotid surgery. Reduction in rSO2 of more than 10 % is regarded as abnormal, the same applies to cerebral ischemia (1, 2, 4, 6, 7).

The regional cerebral oxymetry is a measure of the percentage saturation in the brain's vascular bed. It is a sensitive parameter for determining the relation between oxygen supply and oxygen consumption in the brain. Due to the effect of predominantly venous blood in the cerebral vascular bed, the oxygen saturation measured primarily represents the cerebral venous circulation (4, 6). Apart from the cerebral regional oxygen saturation (rSO2), the somatosensory evoked potentials were registered. We used SEP as a reference method because of the known high reliability. Within the framework of a previous study,

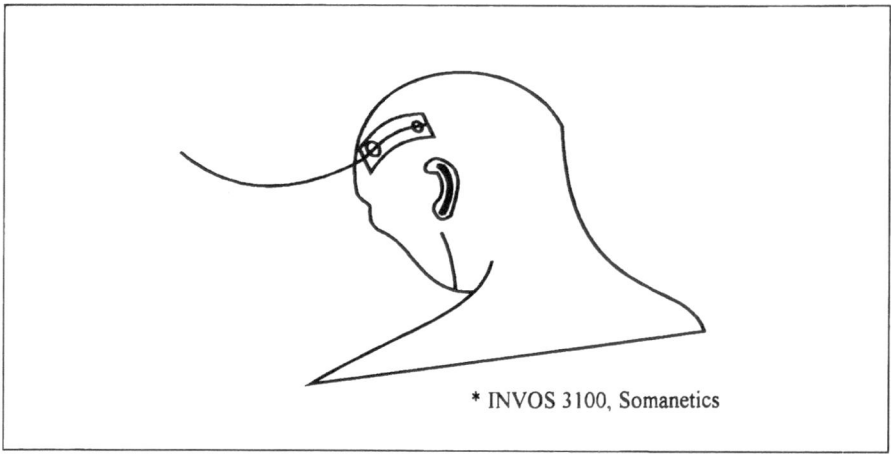

Fig. 1. Regional cerebral oxymetry (RCO) – sensor placement and schematic representation of the tissue layers

we defined that a reduction in the SEP amplitude of more than 50 % was an abnormal finding, and we found a sensitivity of 100 % and specificity of about 90 % using this method (3). After stimulation of the median nerve, we register the evoked potentials from the ipsilateral cortex during carotid surgery, particulary during the clamping period. The N20/P25 amplitude was judged.

From February to September 1994 we studied 136 patients, who underwent 148 carotid endarterectomies. The mean age was 67 years (range 50–81). There were 82 men and 54 women. The indication for carotid endarterectomy was the symptomatic stage (TIA or stroke) in 82 cases. About 80 % of cases showed over 70 % carotid stenosis. In four cases we registered transient ischemic attacks. Three of these patients suffered a transient ischemic attack intraoperatively. Another patient showed a neurological deficit lasting a few hours during the observation period in the intensive care unit due to a hypertensive crisis. We observed intraoperative stroke with remaining neurological deficits in only one case.

The statistical analysis found a sensitivity of 66.6 % and a specificity of 97.7 %. The positive and negative predictive value was 80 % and 95.5 % (Table 1). Four cases showed abnormal cerebral oxygen saturation and somatosensory evoked potentials. In these

Table 1. Sensitivity, specifity, and predictive value (PV) of the transcranial oxymetry as a monitoring device during carotid surgery

		abnormal oxymetry	
		yes	no
abnormal SEP	yes	12	3
	no	6	127

sensitivity: 66,6 %   pos. PV: 80,0 %
specificity: 97,7 %   neg. PV: 95,5 %

cases, we inserted an intraluminal shunt. The rate of shunting was 9.3 % (n = 4). Despite shunting one of these patients suffered an intraoperative neurological deficit such as a TIA. In this case the abnormal monitorings were observed seven minutes after cross-clamping. Both control methods showed a slow normalization of values after shunt insertion. In three other cases the oxygen saturation of brain and somatosensory evoked potentials of the ipsilateral cortex were abnormal, too. The postoperative course of these patients was free of complications. The clamping period was less than 3 minutes.

Fig. 2 shows sequential cerebral oxygen changes during the important phases of the operation. After clamping the carotid artery, the oxygen saturation is usually reduced by about 5–8 %. At the end of the operation we often see a short-term increase of the rSO2 because cerebral re-perfusion. The abnormal oxymetry is demonstrated in Fig. 3. After the clamping the oxygen saturation is always reduced more than 10 %. After the placement of an intraluminal shunt, we see a clear increase of saturation. In all abnormal cases we did not notice the complete normalization of oxymetry, but at the end of clamping, we registered a complete normalization. The short-term increase of oxygen saturation is also observed in these situations.

Discussion

The risk of cerebral ischemia during the clamping period is always present during carotid endarterectomy. In agreement with most vascular surgeons we consider intraoperative monitoring is important and a necessity. The existing methods with an established high

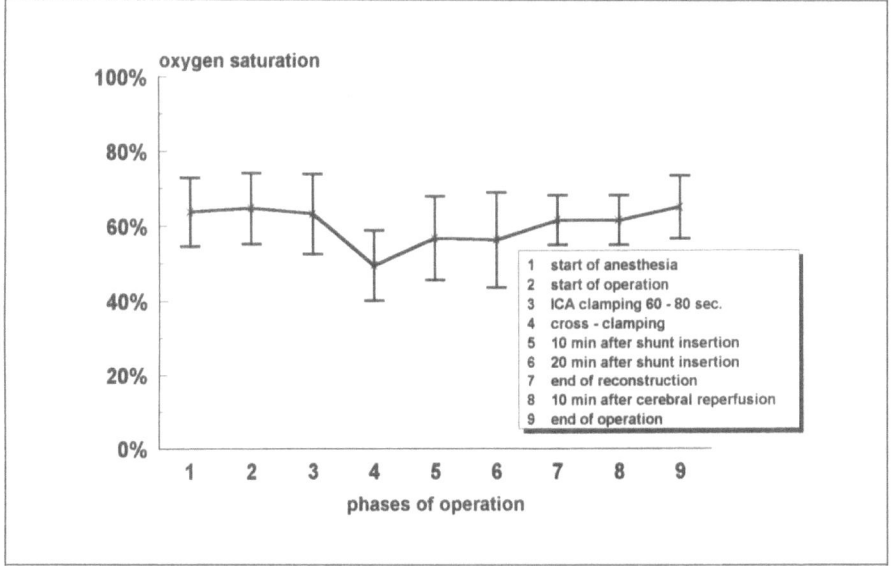

Fig. 2. Abnormal change (more than 10 %) of cerebral oxygen saturation during carotid clamping (n = 18)

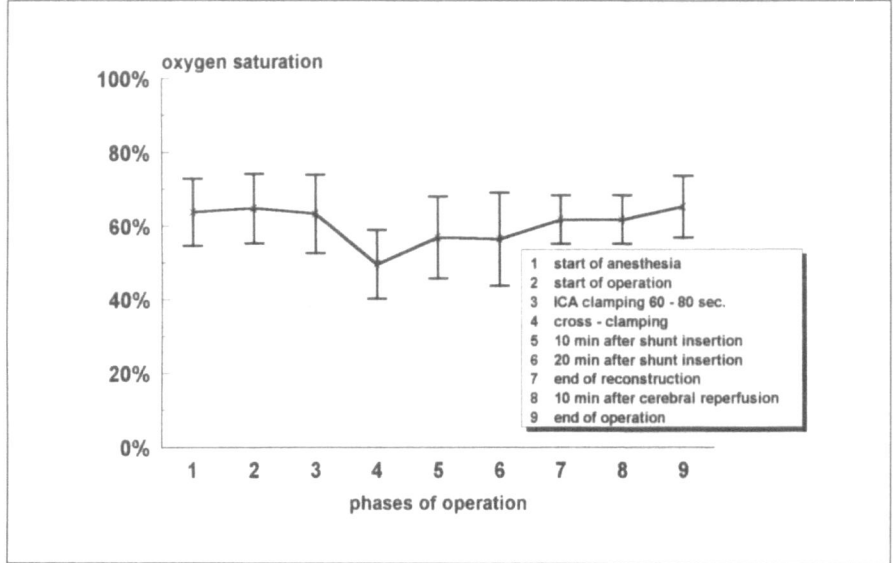

Fig. 3. Non-significant reduction of cerebral oxygen saturation during carotid operation (n = 130)

reliability are the somatosensory evoked potentials (SEP) and electroencephalography (EEG). Alternatively, the surgery under local or regional anesthesia is also possible (3, 5, 6).

The cerebral regional oxygen saturation seems to be an additional useful monitor in carotid surgery. If good reliability is confirmed in the further course of our study, we predict a very quick establishment of this method. Other reasons for increased popularity are the simplicity of the method and no additional personnel requirement.

Further advantages were the non-invasive technique and the continuity of monitoring. In contrast to the other established methods (SEP, EEG), this technique shows a favorable cost/effectiveness relationship (6).

References

1. Cairns CB, Fellipo D, Proctor HJ (1985) Non-invasive method for monitoring the effects of increased intracranial pressure with near infrared spectrophotometry. Surg Gynecol Obstet 196: 145–8
2. Ferrari M, Zanette E, Sideri G, Giannini I, Fieschi C (1987) Effects of carotid compression as assessement by near infrared spectroscopy upon cerebral blood volume and hemoglobin oxygen. J Royal Soc Med 80: 83–87
3. Horsch S, De Vleeschauwer P, Ktenidis K (1990) Intraoperative assessment of cerebral ischemia during carotid surgery. J Cardiovasc Surg 31: 599
4. McCormick PW, Stewart M, Goetting MG, Dujovny M, Lewis G, Ausman JI (1991) Non-invasive cerebral optical spectroscopy for monitoring cerebral delivery and hemodynamics. Critical Care Medicine 19: 89–97
5. Panetta TF (1995) Somatosensory evoked potential monitorring, carotid stump pressure and the status of the contralateral carotid artery as indicators for shunting: Which is the best In: Current Crytucal Problems, New Horizons and Techniques in Vascular and Endovascular Surgery. Frank J. Veith (Symposiums Chairman), New York

6. Williams IM, McCollum C (1993) Cerebral oxymetry in carotid endarterectomy and acute stroke. In: Greenhalgh RM, Hollier LH (eds) Surgery for Stroke. WB Saunders Company Ltd, London, 129–38
7. Wray S, Cope M, Delipy DI, Wyatt JS, Reynolds EOR (1988) Characterization of the near infrared absorption spectra of cytochrome aa3 and hemoglobin for the non-invasive monitoring of cerebral oxygenation. Biochem et Biophys Acta 993: 184–92

Author's address:
Kiriakos Ktenidis, MD
Krankenhaus Porz am Rhein,
Teach.-Hospital of Univ. of Cologne
Department of General and Vascular Surgery
Urbacher Weg 19
51149 Köln, Germany

Polytetrafluoroethylene (PTFE) interposition graft in carotid surgery: indications and late results

I. Mogán, L. Entz[1], D. Raithel[2]

Budai MÁV Hospital Vascular Surgery
1 Cardiovascular Surgical Clinic of Semmelweis Medical University,
2 Klinikum Nürnberg Department of Vascular Surgery

The surgical techniques of carotid endarterectomy have been widely discussed by vascular surgeons and neurosurgeons. All experts of carotid surgery agree on the importance of carefully performed endarterectomy and meticulous cleaning of the endarterectomized surface of the carotid bifurcation and internal carotid artery (ICA) to avoid thrombembolic complications. However, there is a significant difference in the opinions of different authors about the technique of the arterial closure after endarterectomy. We think that there are some situations in which the endarterectomy and any types of arterial closure would be very difficult or even impossible to perform, such as in the presence of aneurysms, or dilatations of the bifurcation (Fig. 1), tortuosities involving long segment of ICA, highly extended atherosclerotic lesions with exulcerations (Fig. 2), or in some special cases of reccurent carotid stenosis. We have been using thin-walled PTFE prosthesis to reconstruct such lesions since 1984 in Budapest (A) (1), and since 1985 in Nuremberg (B). We have studied the perioperative and late results of these operations in both centers to determine its efficacy and the long-term clinical outcome.

Material and method

A) At the Cardiovascular Surgical Clinic, Semmelweis Medical University of Budapest a total of 1123 carotid operations were performed between Jan. 1, 1984 and Dez. 31, 1991. During this period 42 (3.7 %) PTFE interposition grafts were implanted. Our sample included 27 men and 15 women with a mean age of 62.5 years (42 – 84 yrs). In 17 cases the right and in 25 the left internal carotid arteries were reconstructed. Six-mm thin-walled PTFE grafts were used in all but two operations, in which 5-mm, prosthesis were implanted to obtain a proper size match with the internal carotid artery.

In 83 % of cases intraluminal shunt was used. Mean clamping time of the internal carotid artery was 47 min (24 – 58 min). The indications for PTFE interpositions are summarized in Table 1. The perioperative neurological stages of the patients were as follows, asymptomatic: 1. TIA/amaurosis fugax; 17, progressive stroke, early postoperative complications after TEA or EEA of ICA; 12, completed stroke; 7, nonhaemispheric symptoms; 5 cases.

B) During a period of 6 years (Jan. 1, 1985 – Dez. 31, 1991) 5122 carotid artery reconstructions were performed in Klinikum Nuremberg Department of Vascular Surgery. From this material 71 interpositions (1.4 %) were implanted (42 PTFE-29 great saphenous vein). This sample included 49 men and 22 women with a mean age of 66.2 years (48 – 82

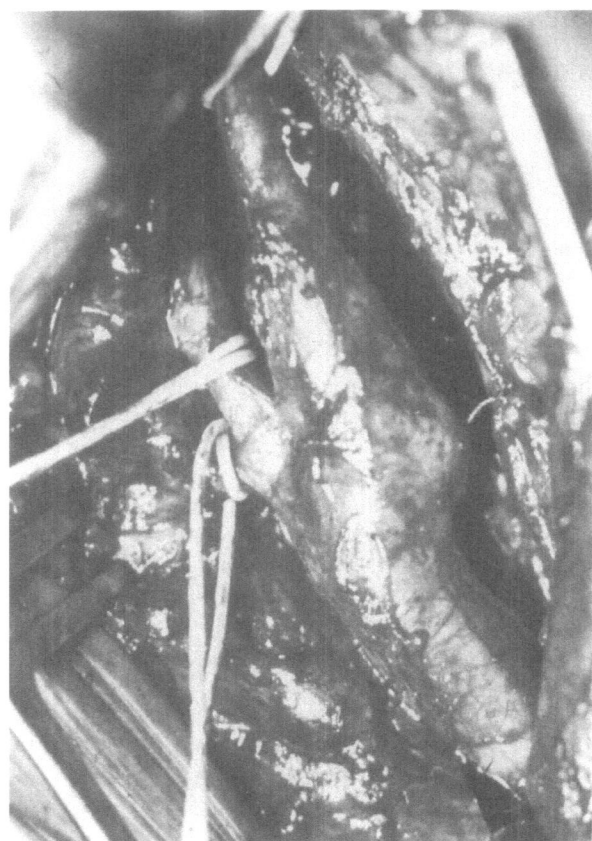

Fig. 1. Dilated carotid bifurcation.

Table 1. Indication for PTFE interposition graft (Budapest)

	Number of cases
Long-segment stenosis of ICA with exulceration or dilatation	7
Severe tortuosity of ICA with stenosis	14
Aneurysm of ICA/CCA	3
Recurrent stenosis of ICA	2
Technical problem during endarterectomy of ICA	4
Early postoperative thrombosis of ICA	12

years). Intraluminal shunt was not used The mean clamping time was 42.3 min (22 – 53 min). The indications for interpositions are shown in Table 2. The preoperative neurological stages were as follows, asymptomatic: 11, TIA/amaurosis fugax; 25, completed stroke; 17, progressive stroke; 18 cases.

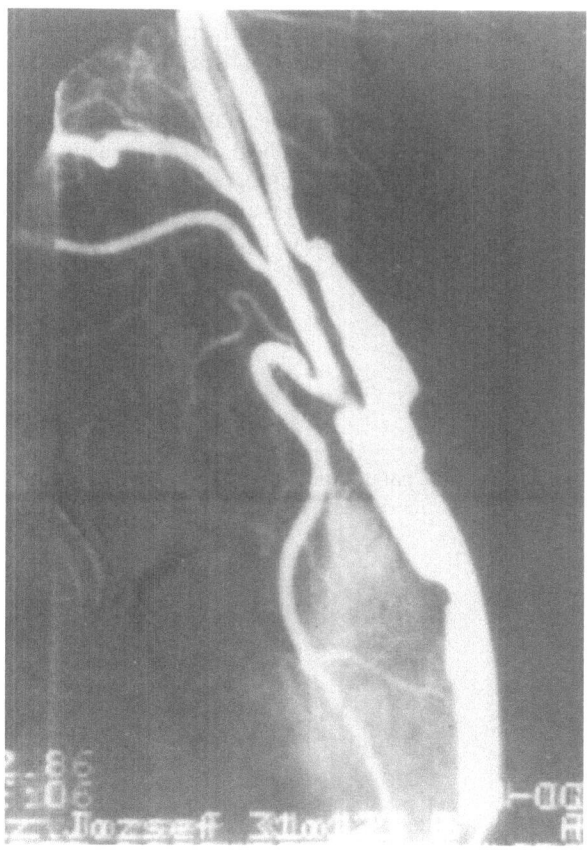

Fig. 2. Atherosclerotic lesion with exulcerations, extended on a long segment of common, external and internal carotid artery.

Table 2. Indication for interposition graft (Nuremberg)

	PTFE	VEIN
Long-segment stenosis of ICA with exulceration	2	7
Severe tortuosity of ICA	3	1
Aneurysm of ICA	2	1
Recurrent stenosis	7	3
Patch aneurysm	3	–
Technical problem during EEA/TEA	19	1
Late infections after Dacron patch	–	6
Early postoperative thrombosis	6	11
Postoperative bleeding	–	1

Operative technique: in general anesthesia conventional approach of the carotid bifurcation. The involved segment of the internal carotid artery is resected and a 6-mm diameter thin-walled PTFE prosthesis is obliquely anastomosed to the cranial stump of ICA at first. Having finished this anastomosis the internal carotid artery is dilated. The common and external carotid arteries are conventionally endarterectomised and after this a long, oblique proximal anastomosis is performed. Both anastomoses are sewn with continuous monofilament 6/0 polypropylane suture (Fig. 3).

Follow-up was performed by duplex scan every 6 months. A general follow-up was made in Nuremberg in May 1992 and in Budapest in 1995 with the help of questionnaire, personal consultation and duplex scan. Digital substraction arteriography (DSA) was performed whenever hemodynamically significant recurrent stenosis or contralateral stenosis was detected on duplex scan. Aspirin was routinely administered.

Results

A) There were three perioperative deaths. One patient died on the second postoperative day because of myocardial infarction. She was operated on because of ruptured aneurysm

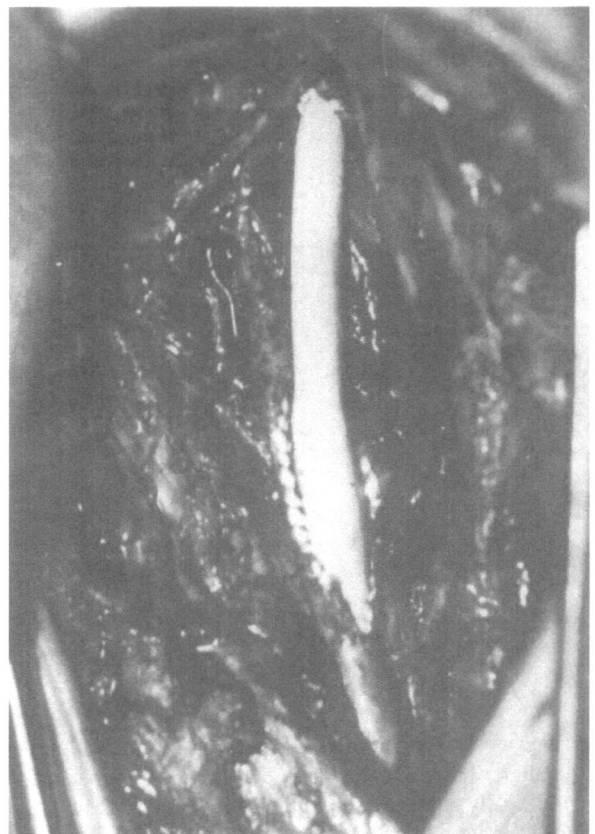

Fig. 3. PTFE interposition graft between the bifurcation and the internal carotid artery.

of the carotid bifurcation. The other two patients initially were operated on with eversion technique and in the early postoperative period the endarterectomised segment thrombotized. Both patients were operated in stage of fulminant progressive stroke. After the second operation (PTFE interposition) the patients remained unconscious and died on the third and fourth postoperative day, respectively. New permanent neurological symptoms after interposition graft were not observed; one TIA occurred. One patient with postoperative bleeding was reoperated with success. One graft reoccluded on the third postoperative day, the patient developed nonhemisphaeric symptoms.

The mean follow-up period was 56 months (38 – 120 months). We have lost seven patients from the follow-up. Ten patients died; the causes of death were as follows: two strokes (one ipsilateral, one contralateral), five myocardial infarctions, three unknown. One patient had ipsilateral stroke caused by thrombosis of the implanted PTFE graft 50 months postoperatively. Based on duplex scanning 18 interposition grafts were patent, in three cases mild restenosis (< 50 %), in one patient a significant stenosis (asymptomatic) were found. We have observed neither infections nor aneurysm formations.

B) In all patients who were operated on in the stage of progressive stroke the indication for interposition graft was reocclusion or rethrombosis after conventional or eversion endarterectomies of ICA. Three patients died of stroke, eight patients had hemisymptomatic after the interposition graft and 60 patients had good recovery and were symptomfree at discharge from the hospital. In five patients TIA was observed. Because of postoperative haematoma three patients were reoperated. One patient had an infection after a vein graft implantation and was treated conservatively. Early reocclusion was not observed. One patient had a fatal myocardial infarction.

Follow-up was obtained in all but one patient and ranged from 6 to 84 months with a mean of 18 (PTFE group) and 25 (vein group) months, respectively. Every 6 months a duplex scan was performed and in 26 patients DSA was done. The follow-up data are summarized in Table 3.

One patient in the vein group was reoperated because of the development of a significant symptomatic restenosis and a new PTFE interposition graft was implanted after excision of the vein graft.

Table 3. Late results after interposition graft (Nuremberg)

	PTFE	VEIN
Restenosis < 50 %	3	1
Restenosis > 50 %	1	3
Anastomosis dilatation	–	2
Late infection	–	–
Reocclusion	–	–
Asymptomatic	30	11
TIA (ipsilateral)	–	2
Permanent neurological deficit	3	6
Stroke: ipsilateral	–	1
- contralateral	1	2
Death	2	3

Discussion

After complicated endarterectomies of the carotid bifurcation the arterial closure can be difficult or unsafe, especially in cases in which tortuosity or long-segment stenosis are present. Using eversion endarterectomy, in some instances the distal intima cannot be fixed and the floating edge of the intima can lead to thrombembolic complications (Fig. 4). The arterial wall is very thin after endarterectomy of intramural calcifications and in case of hypertension it can rupture in the early postoperative period. These problems can be easily prevented by the interposition technique (1 – 6).

On the basis of our 10-year experience, we consequently apply the interposition method with the following indications:

In elective cases

In the presence of *long-segment stenosis with exulceration and/or dilatation* of the internal carotid artery: In such cases the intima fixation and patch plasty with sufficient overpass

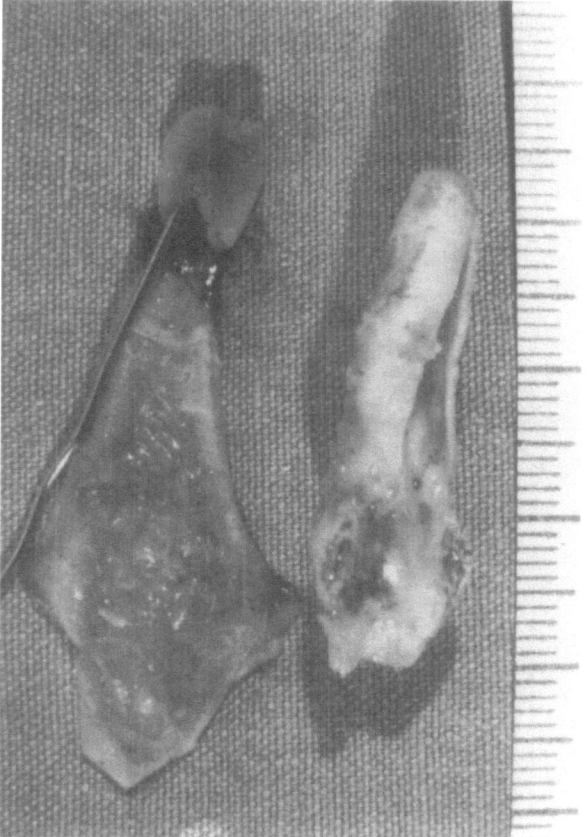

Fig. 4. Failed eversion endarterectomy of the internal carotid artery. The distal intima edge is ruptured and cannot be fixed. The involved segment is resected.

can be very difficult or even impossible. It is simpler and safer to resect the involved segment and to implant either autogenous vein or prosthetic graft.

Complicated tortuosity of ICA

There are some well known techniques to eliminate the kinks or coilings, but if a torquation is also present all these methods will fail, because neither the implication technique nor the reimplantation method are suitable to ensure a sufficient detorquation of the internal carotid artery. Resection of the diseased segment and implantation of a graft is the method of choice in these cases.

Recurrent stenosis of ICA

The classical techniques for carotid endarterectomies can be seldom followed in cases of recurrent stenosis because of the changed circumstances, the layers of the plaque are adherent, the adventitia is in scar tissue so a correct exposure of the arteries and the performance of endarterectomy in a convenient layer is not always possible. The interposition technique offers the chance for reconstruction with the lowest rate of complication, although Sise has found a higher percentage of recurrent stenosis in such cases (3). Treiman and others have also reported good results with interposition technique in cases of recurrent stenosis (3, 4, 7, 8).

Patch aneurysms

A rare complication of the patch plasty is aneurysm formation with or without rupture. Because of the dilated and thin-walled bifurcation a partial resection and direct suture is seldom beneficial, so a total resection of the involved area and implantation of an interposition graft remains the one possibility to restore the circulation.

   In such cases the external carotid artery cannot always be saved.

Aneurysms of internal or common carotid arteries

From among the various techniques being used in the surgery of carotid aneurysms, the interposition method is recommended in cases of aneurysms involving a long segment of the internal and/or common carotid arteries (9 – 11).

   In the presence of mycotic aneurysms or with any signs of infection, in spite of one successful case reported (12), the autologous vein is the graft of choice.

Tumors

An extensive involvement of the carotid arteries by any type of tumor including carotid body tumor, may require resection of the arteries and graft interposition (13 – 15).

Intraoperative indication in case of failed eversion endarterectomy or conventional endarterectomy

Using the eversion method for carotid endarterectomy in few cases (1 – 2 % in our material) the safe control of the distal intima is not always possible. In such instances the interposition graft gives the solution.

In these cases the PTFE prosthesis has a particular advantage over the vein because of its prompt availability.

In acute cases

Early postoperative reocclusions

After any type of carotid reconstruction early thrombosis can occur. The causes leading to this severe complication are different, but what is common in them is the thrombogenic surface of the endarterectomized segment (Fig. 5).

The best way to avoid a second thrombosis of ICA is to resect the whole endarterectomized part of ICA and replace it with graft.

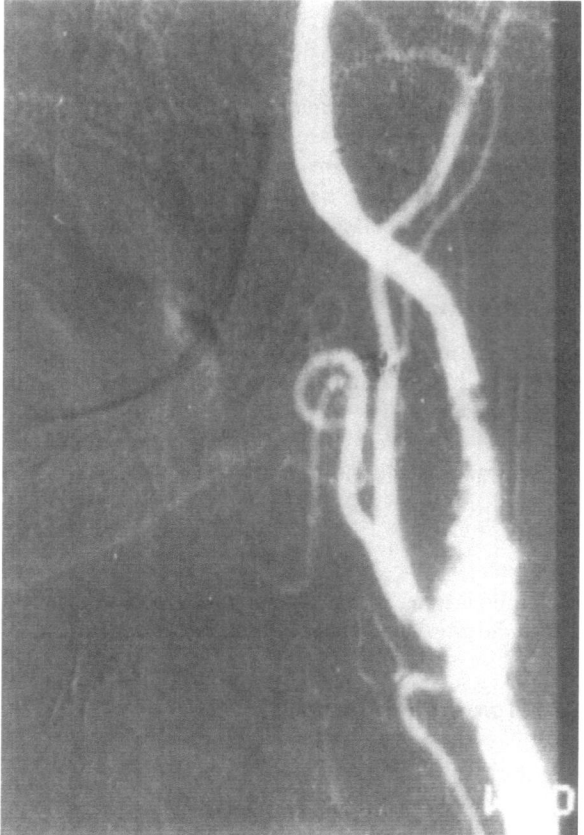

Fig. 5. DSA picture of a partially thrombosed carotid bifucation 2 h after eversion endarterectomy.

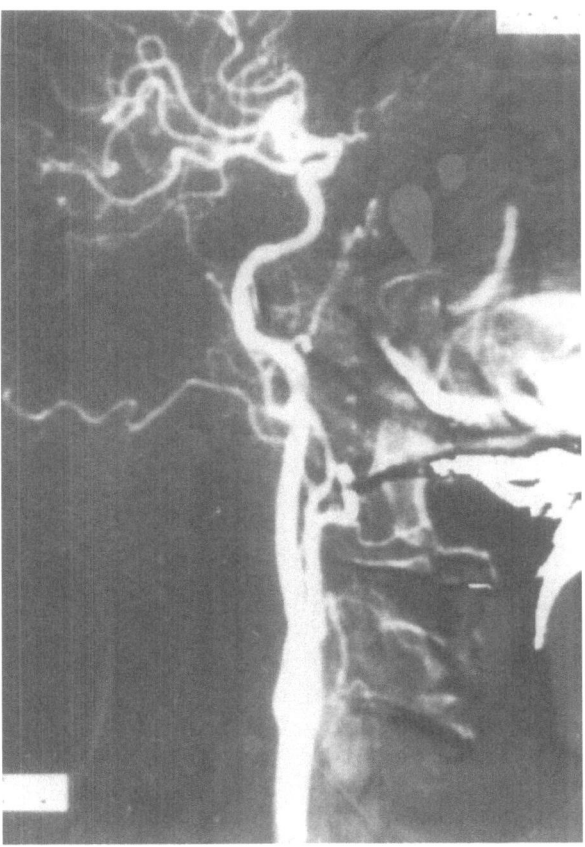

Fig. 6. Control DSA of a PTFE interposition graft implanted 5 years earlier (lateral view).

Ruptured carotid aneurysms

In case of this very rare complication the fastest and safest solution is not to try to restore the ruptured part of ICA, but to resect it, followed by implantation of a graft.

Carotid dissection

Surgery is indicated for every localized carotid dissection, most of them can be treated with excision of the involved segment and graft replacement.

Taking into consideration the early and late results of both centers, we conclude that the interposition method using vein or PTFE prosthesis according to the indications listed above and published in the literature is a safe procedure and sometimes the only method of choice in the surgery of the carotid bifurcation.

We do not want to suggest to that either vein or PTFE prosthesis be preferentially applied for interposition, but we do think that both kind of grafts are conveniert for interposition procedures. Cormier has proposed to use PTFE prosthesis only, when no suitable saphenous vein is available (6). The long-term patency rate of the PTFE grafts proven by

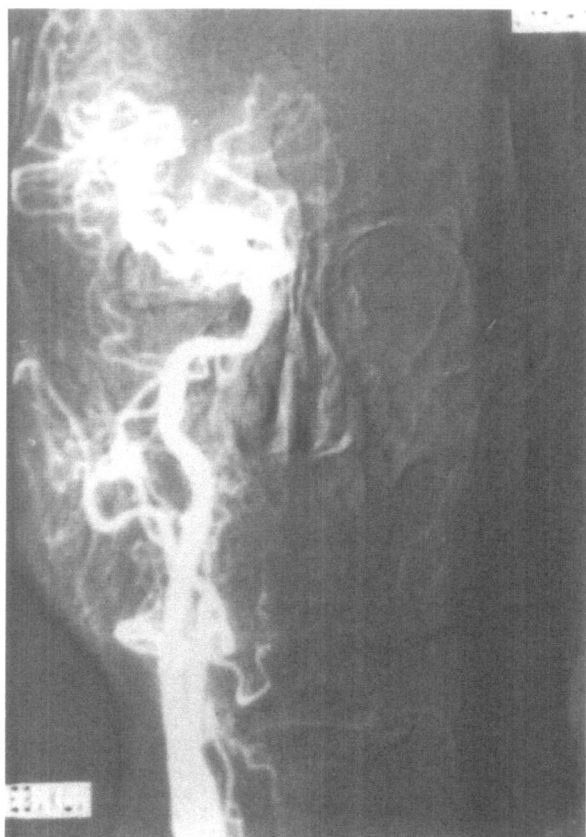

Fig. 7. Control DSA of the same patient (see Fig. 6) from antero-posterior view.

our follow up studies in both centers convinced us to employ the PTFE graft as first choice (Figs. 6, 7).

References

1. Mogán I, Dzsinich CS, Entz L, Papp S, Nemes A (1988) Die Interna Interposition als Alternative einer TEA in der Karotis Chirurgie. Angio Archiv 16: 161–62
2. Thompson JE (1979) Complications of Carotid Endarterectomy and Their Prevention. World J Surg 3: 155–165
3. Sise MJ, Ivy ME, Malanche R, Ranbarger KR (1992) Polytetrafluoroethylene interposition grafts for carotid reconstruction. J Vasc Surg 16: 601–8
4. Gagne JP, Riles TS, Jacobowitz GR, Lamparello PJ, Giangola G, Adelman MA, Imparato AM, Mintzer R (1993) Long-term follow-up of patients undergoing reoperation for recurrent carotid artery disease. J Vasc Surg 18: 991–1001
5. Archie JP (1993) Carotid endarterectomy with reconstruction techniques tailored to operative findings. J Vasc Surg 17: 141–51

6. Cormier JM,Cormier F, Laurian C, Gigou F, Fichelle JM, Bokobza B (1987) Polytetrafluoroethylene bypass for revascularization of the atherosclerotic internal carotid artery: late results. Ann Vasc Surg 1: 564–71
7. Treiman GS, Jenkins JM, Edwards WH, Barlow W, Edwards Jr WH, Martin RS, Mulherin JL (1992) The evolving surgical management of recurrent carotid stenosis. J Vasc Surg 16: 354–363
8. Meyer FB, Piepgras DG, Fode NC (1994) Surgical treatment of recurrent carotid artery stenosis. J Neurosurg 80: 781–7
9. Redaelli C, Carrel T, Turina M (1991) Die Chirurgie der extrakraniellen Aneurysmen der Arteria carotis. Analyse von 8 Fällen. Chirurg 62: 620–4
10. Destian S, Tung H, Gray R, Hinton DR, Day J, Fukushima T (1994) Giant infectious intracavernous carotid artery aneurysm presenting as intractable epistaxis. Surg Neurol 41: 472–6
11. Hamada Y, Inoue T, Hitotsumatsu T, Matsuno H, Imamura H, Ohnishi H (1994) Symptomatic bilateral extracranial internal carotid artery. Fukuoka-Igaku-Zasshi 85: 128–32
12. Pasic M, Schwitter J, Vogt M, Carrel T, Segesser L, Turina M (1992) Ruptured Mycotic Extracranial Carotid Aneurysm Treated by Excision, PTFE Graft Interposition, and Local Antibiotic Application. A Case Report. Vascular Surgery 26: 421–425
13. Meleca RJ, Marks SC (1994) Carotid artery resection for cancer of the head and neck. Arch Otolaryngology 120: 974–8
14. Laube HR, Fahrenkamp AG, Bocker W, Scheld HH (1994) Glomustumoren: eine diagnostische und chirurgische Herausforderung? Z Kardiol 83: 373–80
15. Rabl H, Friehs I, Gutschi S, Pascher O, Koch G (1993) Diagnosis and treatment of carotid body tumors. Thorac Cardiovasc Surg 41: 340–3

Author's address:
J. Mogán, M.D.
Dep. of Vascular Surgery
Budai MAV Hospital
1528 Budapest, Szanatoriumu 2/aa
Hungary

Exclusive PTFE patch angioplasty after conventional carotid endarterectomy: short- and long-term results

W. Reifenhäuser, K. Ktenidis, S. Ricke, S. Horsch

Krankenhaus Porz am Rhein, Department of General and Vascular Surgery, Cologne, Germany

After a long period of up and downs, carotid surgery has become, not least due to the results of recent multicentre studies (1, 2), a worldwide established procedure in preventing cerebro-vascular accidents. The history of carotid surgery is accompanied by controversies about the indications and the operation technique and in most issues no definite answer is found.

The way of arteriotomy closure also continues to be controversial, although several studies revealed a significant benefit in restenosis rates for patch angioplasty (3, 4). Also the reduction of early thrombosis rates was reported by various authors. Nevertheless patching or not patching remains an individual decision as well as the choice of the patch material. Initially an autologous vein, saphenous as well as internal jugular, was used predominantly as patch material. The varied resistance to mechanical stress of the autologous vein may lead to fatal patch rupture (5) or false aneurysm formation. This drawback can be avoided by the use of synthetical patch materials, which provide a constant tensile strength and preserves the saphenous vein for peripheral arterial or aortocoronary bypass procedures. On the other hand the use of synthetical patches may be attached to a higher risk of infection (6) and contributes to the problem of suture hole bleeding.

Early postoperative narrowing of the internal carotid artery after direct suturing is often due to small vessel diameter, while this problem after patch angioplasty is mostly generated by technical faults at the proximal or distal anastomosis or by kinking caused by elongation of the endarterectomied artery.

Materials and methods

In our clinic from January 1986 to August 1994 we performed 2441 carotid endarterectomies including 1374 with polytetrafluorethylene (PTFE) patch angioplasty. We observed the patients prospectively for answers to following questions: the rate of neurological complications; perioperative morbidity and mortality; and the rate of recurrent stenosis. Due to our experience with direct arteriotomy closure and venous patch plasty, we switched step by step to the exclusive use of PTFE patch material.

We perform carotid surgery under general anaesthesia and use sensory evoked potentials (SEP) for cerebral monitoring. If SEP shows significant impair a shunt will be inserted. Application of heparin and use of a suction drainage are mandatory. Follow-up data were gained with bidirectional Doppler sonography and B-mode ultrasound. In case of recurrent stenosis or aneurysmal dilatation angiographic assessment was done.

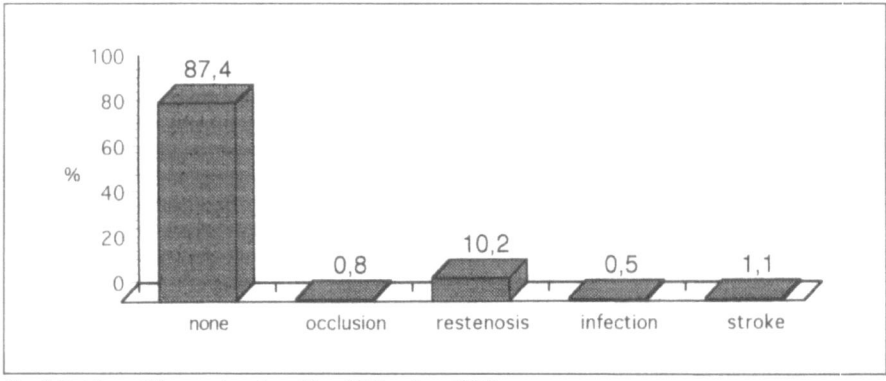

Fig. 1. Total carotid reconstructions (Jan. 1986 – Aug. 1994)

Results

We analysed 1374 carotid endarterectomies with PTFE patch angioplasty performed in 1237 patients. The mean age was 67 years. The follow-up time was 28 months with a range of 1–80 months.

In more than 87 % no complications occurred. Early or late occlusion were observed in 12 patients (0.8 %), the total rate of stenosis > 50 % was 10.2 % (140 patients), in 12 patients (0.8 %) within the first 3 month postoperatively. But only 37 patients (2.7 %) required reoperation for high grade recurrent stenosis with > 70 % narrowing. Deep wound infection was present in 0.5 % (8 patients). A stroke with permanent neurological deficit was observed in 15 patients (1.1 %). Combined perioperative morbidity and mortal-

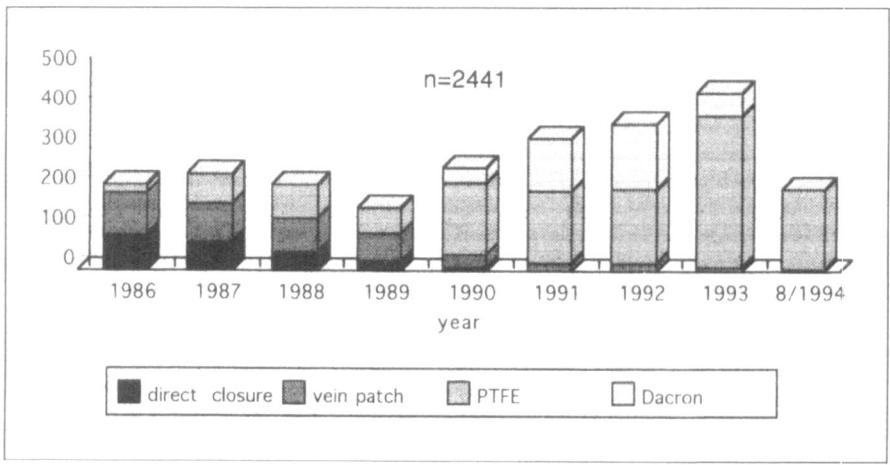

Fig. 2. Complication rates

ity rate of the complete series amount to 3 %; 7 deaths are related to aortic surgery after carotid endarterectomy.

Conclusions

The controversy about carotid surgery still remains. Every argument against operative treatment of high grade stenosis of internal carotid artery will be meaningless, if morbidity and mortality rates are low. In the operation technique the advantages of patch angioplasty seem to exceed direct closure (7, 8). Although there is no consensus in the choice of patch material, the use of synthetic patches, especially polytetrafluorethylene, seems to consistently prevail. The constant and durable quality is able to eliminate an incalculable risk factor. Although, since this year we prefer eversion-endarterectomy, PTFE patch plasty remains a secure and well tried method in carotid surgery, associated with low morbidity, low mortality and an acceptable rate of restenosis, which still has to be proved by other techniques.

References

1. NASCET Collaborators (1991) Beneficial effect of carotid endarterectomy in symptomatic patients with high-grade carotid stenosis. N Engl J Med 325: 445–453
2. The Casanova study group (1991) Carotid surgery versus medical therapy in asymptomatic carotid stenosis. Stroke 22: 1229–1235
3. Katz MM, Jones TG, Degenhardt J et al. (1987) The use of patch angioplasty to alter the incidence of carotid restenosis following thrombendarterectomy. J Cardiovasc Surg 28: 2–8
4. De Letter JAM, Mol FL, Welten RJT et al. (1994) Benefits of carotid patching: a prospective randomized study with long-term followup. Ann Vasc Surg 8: 54–58
5. O'Hara PJ, Hertzer NR, Krajewski LP et al. (1990) Saphenous vein patch rupture after carotid endarterectomy. Surgery 4: 301–304
6. Szilagyi DE, Smith RF, Elliott JP et al. (1972) Infection in arterial reconstruction with synthetic grafts. Ann Surg 176: 321–333
7. Katz D, Snyder SO, Gandhi RH et al. (1994) Long-term follow up for recurrent stenosis: a prospective randomized study of expanded polytetrafluoroethylene patch angioplasty versus primary closure after carotid endarterectomy. J Vasc Surg 19: 198–203
8. Ouriel K, Green RM (1987) Clinical and technical factors influencing recurrent stenosis and occlusion after carotid endarterectomy. J Vasc Surg 5: 702–706

Author's address:
W. Reifenhäuser, M.D.
Krankenhaus Porz am Rhein
Department of General and Vascular Surgery
Urbacher Weg 19
51149 Cologne, Germany

Dacron versus Polyurethane (PUR) patch angioplasty in carotid surgery

G. Albrecht-Früh, K. Ktenidis, W. Reifenhäuser, S. Horsch

Department of General and Vascular Surgery, Krankenhaus Porz am Rhein, Academic Teach.-Hospital of the University of Cologne, Germany

Since reports of the first successful carotid endarterectomy in the early 1950s (3), considerable controversy has evolved regarding the technique und technique of arteriotomy closure. Multiple authors have advocated the use of patch angioplasty in an attempt to decrease the reported high incidence of recurrent carotid artery stenosis after CEA (1, 5, 8). Equally controversial has been the selection of patch material, with supporters for both autogenous tissue and synthetic patches (7, 9, 10).

One of the important arguments against vein patch harvested from the greater saphenous vein especially from the groin is the availability for other possible graft purposes. On the other hand, there is still hesitancy in using synthetic patches, which has been based on the fear of bleeding through the material, intraluminal thrombosus formation, infection, and increasing incidence of myointimal hyperplasia (4, 11).

Study design

This is a short report about a comparison of two synthetic patch materials in a prospective, randomized, monocenter, clinical controlled trial with 104 patients. Both patch materials, which are not used as common as vein or PTFE, are produced by Braun Melsungen. The Dacron patch named "Uni-Graft" is a coated, knitted double microvelour vascular patch. The polyurethane patch called "Cardio-patch" is a structurally modified polyurethane elastomer with high mechanical compliance, superior suture pullout strength, and little tendency to dilatate.

Surgical technique and evaluation of the patch material

All CEA were performed under general endotracheal anesthesia and full heparinization. An intraluminal shunt was used dependent on SEP changes and after the optional tacking suture the arteriotomy closure was done with a running prolene suture.

After finishing the operation, the surgeons evaluated the applicability of the used patch material by rating the handling at suturing and judging the suture hole bleedings. All complications like neurological deficit permanent or transitoric, reoperation because of haematoma, wound infection, or restenosis were documented. Therefore, the patients were examined 3 to 7 days after reconstruction by a neurologist and a surgeon. After discharge, duplex scanning and physical examination were routinely performed at 6 and 12 months after CEA.

We include just the primary carotid reconstructions and selected patients, who were admitted to have carotid endarterectomy on one side. Pregnancy, emergency operation, and infection in the operation area were reasons to exclude these patients from this study.

Results

Analysis of randomized patients shows a male to female preponderance of 2:1. The mean age was 67.1 ± 8.4 years and approximately half of the patients were between the ages of 60 and 69, and 37 % were 70 years or older.

Recognized risk factors for stroke, such as hypertension, diabetes, prior myocardial infarction, and smoking were balanced between the two groups (Table 1).

The indications for CEA were similar in both groups. Asymptomatic high-graded stenosis (> 80 % luminal diameter narrowing) and hemispheric transient ischemic attacks were the most commonly noted indications for operation in each group (Fig. 1). The suture processing and the bleeding from the suture holes were the two criteria to seize the suitability in the operation process. Suture processing was rated as good or very good for both materials (Fig. 2). Also the bleeding from suture holes was very low (Fig. 3) and always refused transfusion. No operation due to haematoma was performed.

The early studies dealt often with patients who only had symptomatic recurrent stenoses. In this study, routinely a carotid duplex scan was used 6 and 12 months after CEA. When frequencies in carotid duplex scanning were found higher than 4 kilohertz, a suspected internal carotid artery restenosis was examined with color flow ultrasonography and angiography.

Two restenoses after CEA with dacron patch angioplasty (3.8 %) and one occlusion after PUR patch angioplasty (1.9 %) were found in the first year (Table 2). It is well known that the most difficult technical aspect of patch placement is sutering it to the apex of the arteriotomy. So it is not astonishing that most of the restenosis were detected in the distal internal carotid artery. Also, in this study both restenosis were found half a year and one year after CEA at a routine examination at the distal end of the dacron patch. Both

Table 1. Risk factors for stroke.

	Dacron (n = 52)	PUR (n = 52)
AGE (> 75 years)	10	5
Hypertension	23	29
Hypercholesterolemia	19	14
Diabetes mellitus	15	11
Overweight (> Broca + 20 %)	7	11
Smoking	21	17
Myocardial infarction	5	4
CHD	19	23

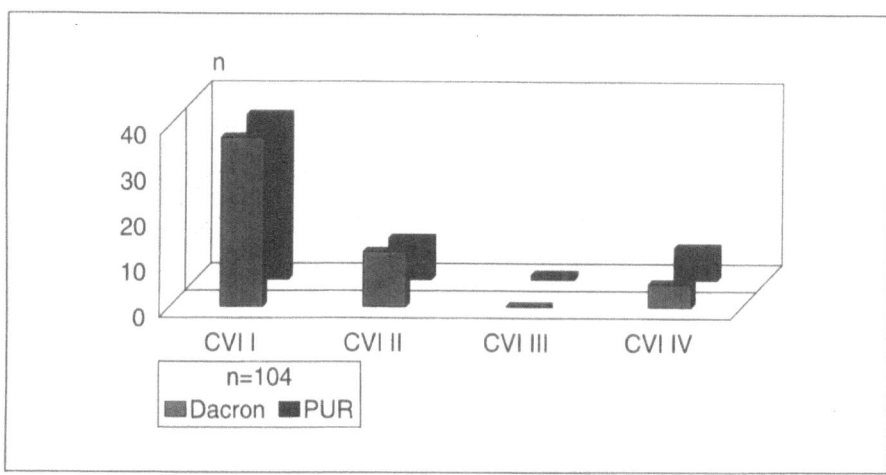

Fig. 1. Preoperative stage and indications.

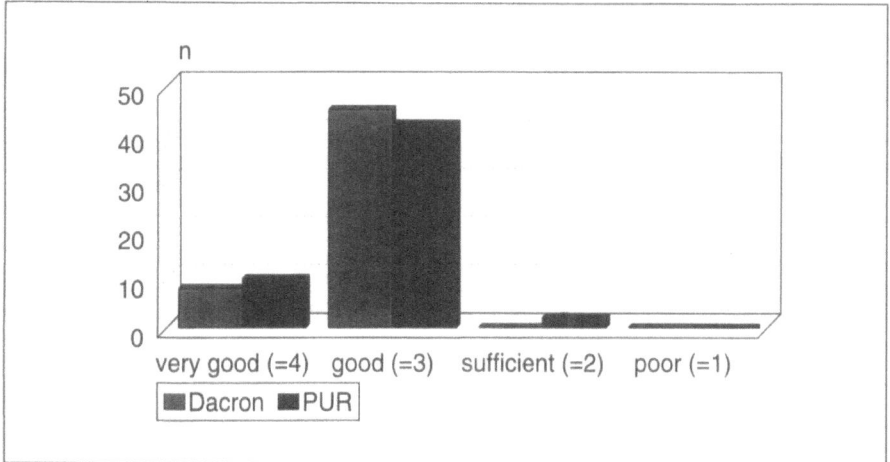

Fig. 2. Valuation of suture processing.

Table 2. Restenoses and occlusion one year after CEA (in %).

	Dacron (n = 52)	PUR (n = 52)	Total (n = 104)
Recurrent stenosis	3.8	0	1.9
Stroke*	0	1.9	1

* after occlusion of internal carotid artery
follow up = 12 months

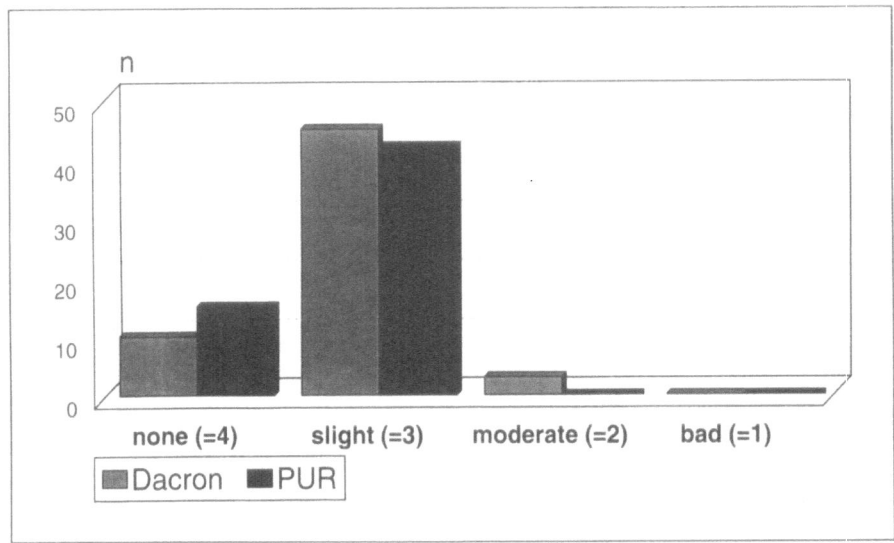

Fig. 3. Valuation of bleeding from suture holes.

patients were asymptomatic and re-endarterectomy and patch angioplasty was performed. No neurological deficit occured perioperatively.

About 2 days after CEA with PUR patch plastic, the 56 year old man developed a symptomatic transitory psychotic syndrom and slight contralateral symptoms. The occlusion of the carotid artery was detected too late that performing a re-operation was impossible; he recovered partially from the stroke.

Two patients died after CEA and patch plastic of a myocardial infarction or a cardial insufficiency perioperativly. The one-year mortality is shown in Table 3. There was one case of delaying wound healing in the PUR group and incompatibility of suture material was supposed. No hint of a deep wound infection or infection of the patch was recognized.

Discussion

The use of a patch to reconstruct CEA is as old as the operation itself and is the mainstay of reconstruction methods used in many series. Although the fact that eversion endar-

Table 3. Mortality perioperative and after one year (in %).

	Dacron (n = 52)	PUR (n = 52)	Total (n = 104)
perioperative mortality	0	3.8*	1.9
mortality one year**	1.9	13.5	7.6
mortality and morbidity perioperative	1.9	3.8	2.8

cause of death: * cardial arrest and infarction; ** 3 myocardial infarctions, 1 accident, 1 carcinoma terectomy is used more frequently and gives the same results in restenosis and occlusion rates even without using a patient's vein or insertion of foreign materials, there are still some recommended indications for selective use of patches. These include ICA diameter less than 3 to 3.5 mm, incomplete or difficult endpoints, repeated operations for recurrent stenosis, and stenosis far above the bifurcation.

Thus, the choice of patch material still remains in question. Although many prefer autologeous tissue, issues have been raised with respect to availability, morbidity related to harvest, patch rupture, late aneurysmal dilatation, and the possible need for these tissues in the future (2). Several studies show no significant difference between saphenous veins and synthetic patches in the early and late restenosis rates (6). Patch rupture is the major concern with CEA patch reconstruction utilizing the greater saphenous vein. Other reasons for not using greater saphenous vein, are leg incision wound problems and the "spare the vein" concept.

The both synthetic patches in this small study showed low suture hole bleedings and good suture processing. There were no problems of biocompatibility and the long-time qualities seem to satisfy the demands of carotid reconstruction.

We have much experience with PTFE patches, as it has been reported. As far as we are concerned it is our opinion that we still need better or improved materials for patches or grafts in vascular reconstruction. And it is necessary to examine new materials to support scientific and marketing development.

References

1. Archie JP (1986) Prevention of early restenosis and thrombosis-occlusion after carotid endarterectomy by saphenous vein patch angioplasty. Stroke 17: 901–905
2. Clagett GP, Rich NM, McDonald PT, Salander JM, Youkey JR, Olson DW, Hutton JE (1983) Etiologic factors for recurrent carotid artery stenosis. Surg 2: 313–318
3. DeBakey ME (1975) Successful carotid endarterectomy for cerebrovascular insufficiency. Jama 233: 1083–1085
4. DeLetter JAM, Moll FL, Welten RJT, Eikelboom BC, Ackerstaff RGA, Vermeulen FEE, Algra A (1994) Benefits of Carotid Patching: A Prospective Randomized study with Long-Term Follow-Up. Ann Vasc Surg 8: 54–58
5. Deriu GP, Ballotta E, Bonavina L et al. (1984) The rationale for patch-graft angioplasty after carotid endarterectomy: early and long-term follow-up. Stroke 15: 972–979
6. Goldman KA, Su WT, Riles TS, Adelman MA, Landis R (1995) A comparative stufy of saphenous vein, internal jugular vein, and knitted Dacron patch for carotid artery endarterectomy. Ann Vasc Surg 9: 71–79
7. Imparato AM (1988) The role of patch angioplasty after carotid endarterectomy. J Vasc Surg 7: 715–716
8. Katz MM, Jones GT, Degenhardt J, Gunn B, Wilson J, Katz S (1987) The use of patch angioplasty to alter the incidence of carotid restenosis following thromboendarterectomy. J Cardiovasc Surg 28: 2–8
9. Katz D, Snyder SO, Gandhi RH, Wheeler JR, Gregory RT, Gayle RG, Parent FN (1994) Longterm follow-up for recurrent stenosis: a prospective randomized study of expanded polytetrafluoroethylene patch angioplasty versus primary closure after carotid endarterectomy. J Vasc Surg 19: 198–205
10. Rhodes VJ (1995) Expanded polytetrafluoroethylene patch angioplasty in carotid endarterectomy. J Vasc Surg 22: 724–731
11. Schmitt DD, Bandyk DF, Pequet AJ, Towne JB (1986) Bacterial adherence to vascular prostheses. J Vasc Surg 3: 732–740

Author's address:
G.-W. Albrecht-Früh
Dept. of General and Vascular Surgery
Academic Teach.-Hospital
University of Cologne
Urbacher Weg 19
51149 Köln, Germany

Eversion versus conventional carotid endarterectomy

K. Balzer

Department of Vascular Surgery (Head: Dr. K. Balzer) of the Evangelical Hospital Muelheim on the Ruhr

Introduction

According to the NASCET Study, the Veterans Administration Study, as well as, the European Study the discussions concerning the indication for an operative treatment of carotid artery stenosis which lasted over years, may be regarded as completed. The impressive results showed that the operative intervention is of less risk for the patient than the natural history. The multicenter studies have been negatively influenced by some high figures from participating centers. Nevertheless, with a percentage clearly lower than 3 % concerning operative morbidity and mortality, the benefit of the vascular surgery can be proved.

In discussing this subject, one fact is frequently omitted: the perioperative risk figure is augmented especially by that group of patients who will not be able to gain any profit by the vascular surgical management due to their advanced stage III or IV which consequently results in a high rate of complications.

Indication for operation

Operative indication should follow careful clinical examinations including the consideration of symptoma. Therefore, noninvasive screening tests, particularly the Doppler-ultrasound-sonography and the Duplex-scanning, are of decisive importance. By means of the Duplex-scanning the morphological diagnosis of arteriosclerosis will be made and so the risk of embolization following soft-plaques can be determined. Apparently, calcified hard-plaques are less dangerous in spite of a high degree stenosis. Angiography may be omitted in cases where the carotid stenosis is unmistakably identified. In the cases of symptomatic carotid stenosis, but usually also in asymptomatic stenosis, a CT-scan for the clarification of unnoticed ischemic insults or the differential diagnosis of a multiinfarct syndrome is indispensable. The transcranial Doppler ultrasound is a proved method for the screening of the collateral perfusion. Age and accompanying diseases are a less important factor for the operative indication.

Operative technique

The surgical approach must follow for good exposure of the arterial region in question. This is best done by an incision made at the anterior margin of the stenocleidomastoid muscle. After sufficient, preparation of the vessels and clamping, a short arteriotomy is made to open the common carotid artery and is extended into the internal carotid artery until an undiseased segment of the artery is reached and the stenotic plug can be visualized and dissected in its entirety. The incision has to be extended far enough into the internal carotid artery, so that a possible resulting distal step from an endarterectomy can be tacked with atraumatic suture to prevent a dissection. Disobliteration often leads to distinct elongation of the vessel if cleavage has taken place between the outer layer of the media and the adventitia. This must be corrected in every case. Endarterectomy of the internal carotid artery is continued into the common carotid artery. If the atheromatous plug with an inner core containing intima and media does not tapper off at its proximal end, it must be sharply divided, leaving a small ledge behind. Retrograde application of the ring stripper may be unsafe and hazardous and will not remove the thickened intima without leaving a ledge or injuring the artery at its origin. In this case the reconstruction must be carried out under proximal preparation under controlled circumstances.

The dissection of the stenotic layer might already be done under the insertion of an intraluminal shunt. The introduction of the shunt enables the reconstruction of the cerebral circulation. Whether or not a shunt should be added is still debated; the results of the teams working without a shunt are not inferior to those who generally use a shunt. In between is the group of elective shunters who make their decision to use a shunt or not depending on evoked potentials, EEG-monitoring with trendanalyser, or transcranial Doppler. We personally only insert a shunt if corresponding changes in the EEG or evoked potentials are seen, or if the transcranial Doppler indicates a critical ischemia or complete occlusion of blood flow in the medial cerebral artery. Great care should be taken not to inflict any injury or embolisation when inserting the shunt. A premature clamping is good protection against peripheral embolisation and better than the disadvantages of long clamping times. All protective measurements formerly undertaken have failed.

The closure of the arteriotomy is usually done with a patch graft. Either an autogenous vein, harvested from the great saphenous vein above the medial malleolus, or a synthetic patch may be used. It also might be done by direct suture, which leads though to a higher restenosis rate. It is of important evidence to review the external carotid artery. Otherwise an occlusion of this vessel may occur. More dangerous is which such a ledge may extend into the internal carotid artery with a postoperative thrombosis.

For some years the new method of the eversion endarterectomy has been available. After transection of the internal carotid artery the adventitial layer is turned upside down over the stenosing plug. It is important to consider adversion of a distal intimal flap. That is why angioscopy after surgical procedure is mandatory to control the lumen of the vessel. More or less long incisions of the arterial stumps allow a shortening of elongations. It is not necessary to implant synthetic material. After early skepticism, the new method has become more and more popular.

Results

Based on a prospective study on 600 patients, we were found remarkable advantages for the eversion technique. Nevertheless, the figures turned out to be too small to prove a statistical significance, but the review of a retrospective analysis on 5000 patients proved the advantages of this method. Therefore, we do believe the eversion endarterectomy is the method of choice whenever possible as opposed to the conventional operative technique.

Concerning the results we would like to refer to the perspectives of the two operative procedures. Irregardless of the selected procedure, the highest risk exists in stage III and IV. The stages I and II indicate a complication rate of less than 2 % in the group of the conventional technique. In the group of eversion endarterectomy, however, we found that none of the patients in these stages died or suffered from a permanent neurological deficit (Tables 1 + 2).

Transitoric neurological disorders with paralytic symptoms, loss of speech, etc. were found in the group of thrombendarterectomy with a rate of 8 %, and in the eversion group a rate of 3 %. These damages disappeared completely after 1 day and are most likely due to the clamping of the cerebral perfusion. The clamping time in the group of the conventional method is about half an hour and in the group of the eversion technique approximately 16 minutes. A correlation between clamping time and postoperative neurological findings is most likely.

In the group of conventional endarterectomy, 9 % had to be reoperated because of postoperative bleedings. This percentage was considerably lower in the eversion group. EEG-changes could be seen more often by conventionally operated patients with a rate of 12.2 % and in the group of the eversion only 4.9 %. A shunt was used in 6.5 % of the conventional cases compared to 2.8 % in the eversion group. Certainly it is more difficult to insert a shunt using the eversion technique (Tables 3 + 4).

A postoperative examination with ultrasound-Doppler und Duplex scanning showed a relatively high figure (11.4 % conventional endarterectomy, 9.2 % eversion endarterectomy) of intimal hyperplasia, which was seen during the first 6 months, but not followed by real recurrent stenoses later on.

The postoperative examination after 6 months shows no essential differences regarding the longterm results of the two different methods. Recurrent stenoses could be proved in 3.8 % of the conventionally operated and in 3.9 % of the eversion group. After one year

Table 1. Carotid surgery trial hospital mortality

	conventional TEA	eversion TEA
stage I	0	0
stage II	1 = 0.5 %	0
stage III	1 = 25 %	0
stage IV	1 = 2.5 %	1 = 2.2 %
total	3/278 = 1.1 %	1/286 = 0.3 %

Table 2. Carotid surgery trial hospital morbidity

	conventional TEA	eversion TEA
stage I	1 = 3.5 %	0
stage II	2 = 1.0 %	0
stage III	1 = 25 %	1 = 33 %
stage IV	2 = 4.3 %	1 = 2.2 %
total	6/278 = 2.2 %	2/286 = 0.6 %

Table 3. Trial on operative technique carotid artery

	convent. TEA	eversion TEA
randomization	blocks of 50	blocks of 50
number	300	300
evaluable	278	286
elongations, dissections, inoperable occlusions	22	14
male/female	64 % / 36 %	68 % / 32 %
age	68.5	64.2
left / right	56 / 44	52 / 48

Table 4. Trial on operative technique carotid artery

	convent. TEA	eversion TEA
revision because of bleeding	24 = 8.6 %	16 = 5.6 %
temporary neurol. disorders	22 = 8 %	7 = 2.5 %
clamping time	28 min	16 min
EEG-changes	34 = 12.2 %	14 = 4.9 %
use of shunt	18 = 6.5 %	8 = 2.8 %
angioscopy	2 = 0.1 %	280 = 98.0 %

less than 1 % in both groups suffered from transitoric ischemic attacks. One stroke occured during the 2 years in the eversion endarterectomy group. According to the life-table analysis 93 % of the TEA-group and 95 % of the eversion group survived the first year with 88 % and 90 %, respectively, in the second year. By omitting the stages III and IV the results improve to 96 % for the first and 92 % for the second year of the two groups. All deaths were due to cardiac failure with the exception of one deadly stroke. Two patients died due to cancer (Fig. 1).

Conclusions

Reasonable results are reported by all experienced centers. It can be noted that surgery on the carotid artery is of significant advantage compared to the conservative therapy, which is always included in the operative treatment. This can be adequately proven by actual studies. By restricting the complications to the stages I and II, they show in our experience a percentage of less than 2 % concerning the conventional technique. No complications were observed by using the eversion endarterectomy in these stages. This underlines not only the advantage of the surgical management in stage II, but also in the asymptomatic stage I. The good results of the eversion endarterectomy point out the benefit of this surgical technique, which should be used whenever possible (Fig. 2). The perioperative monitoring is of high importance. We prefer evoked potentials or the EEG with trend-analyser. Certainly the success of the surgical management depends on the skill and experience of the surgeon. This allows an extended indication of the future when con-

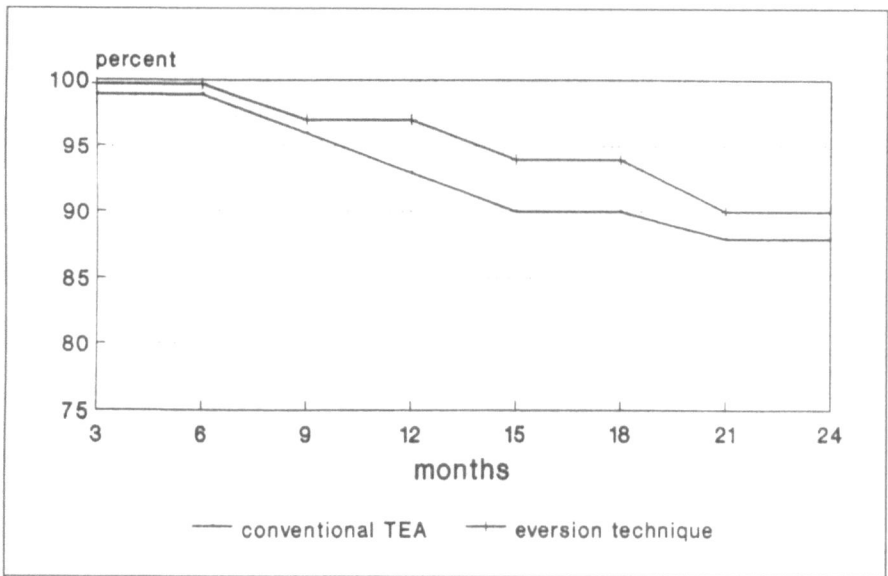

Fig. 1. Lifetable analysis of operative techniques

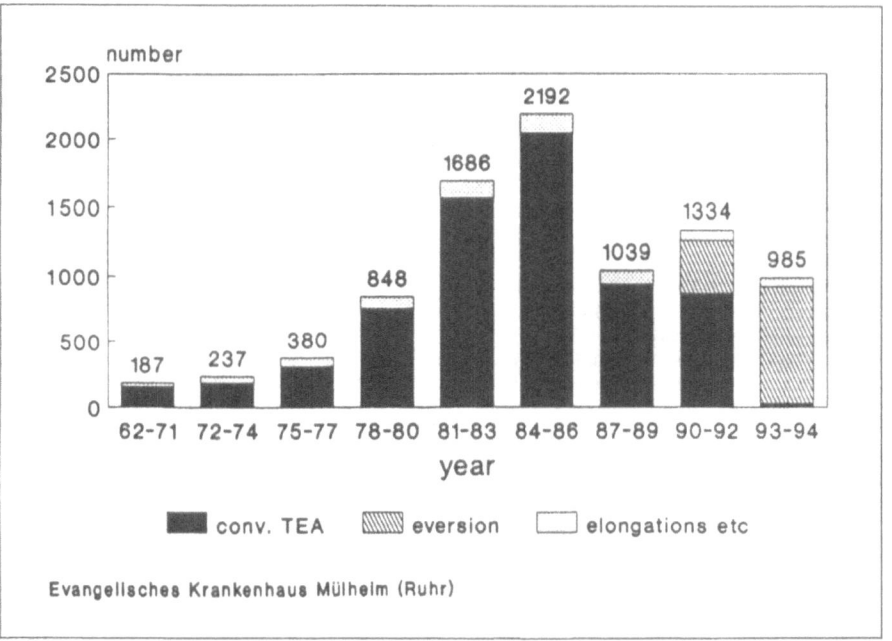

Fig. 2. Surgery on the carotid artery number of operations

siderating Duplex scanning and in regard to the type of the atherosclerotic disease. The long term morbidity and mortality is less in the stages I and II. This points out the importance of timely prophylactic operation. Most patients died because of cardiac failure; stroke is – as seen by this – a rarely seen postoperative complication. The safety of the patient demands a sufficient diagnostic procedure as well as a consequent indication. Both are as important as good surgical and postoperative management.

Karos in the Greek language means heavy sleep. The ancient Greeks called the arteries of the neck "carotid arteries", because they believed that when they were pressed hard, a man became sleepy. According to legend the Centaur fought against a soldier using the technique of pressing the carotid artery. In this way he won the fight. From the vascular surgical point of view, we should do our best that the name for this artery does not represent its meaning. That means fighting against stroke with a safe operative technique and with timely vascular reconstruction.

References

1. Aburahma AF, Robinson P, Decanio R (1989) Prospective clinicopathologic study of carotid intraplaque hemorrhage. Am Surg 55: 169–73
2. Anderson RJ, Hobson RW 2d, Padberg FT Jr, Pecoraro JP, De Groote RD, Jamil Z, Lee BC, Breitbart GB, Franco DC (1991) Carotid endarterectomy for asymptomatic carotid stenosis: a ten year experience with 120 procedures in a fellowship training program. Ann Vasc Surg 5: 111–5
3. Autret A, Saudeau D (1986) Atherome: quelles carotides operer? Presse Med 15: 205–9
4. Balzer K, Carstensen G (1985) Rekonstruktionen an der A. carotis. Ökonomie der Diagnostik und Ergebnisse. DMW 110: 510–512
5. Brott T, Thalinger K (1984) The practice of carotid endarterectomy in a large metropolitan area. Stroke 15: 950–955
6. Caracci BF, Zukowski AJ, Hurley JJ, Naunheim KS, Auer AI (1989) Asymptomatic severe carotid stenosis. J Vasc Surg 9: 361–6
7. Carstensen G, Balzer K (1986) Die asymptomatische Carotisstenose: Wann soll – wann muß man – wann soll man nicht operieren? Langenbecks Arch Chir 369: 97–103
8. Carstensen G, Balzer K (1988) Surgery of the carotid artery. In: Heberer, van Dongen (eds) Vascular Surgery. Springer, Berlin Heidelberg
9. Casanova Study Group (1991) Carotid surgery versus medical therapy in asymptomatic carotid stenosis. Stroke 22: 1229–35
10. Cebul RD, Whisnant JP (1989) Carotid endarterectomy. Ann Intern Med 111: 660–70
11. Chambers BR, Norris JW (1986) The case against surgery for asymptomatic carotid and coronary artery disease. J Vasc Surg 3: 690–2
12. Deruty R, Mottolese C, Pelissou-Guyotat I, Lapras C (1991) The carotid endarterectomy: experience with 260 cases and discussion of the indications. Acta Neurochir Wien 112: 1–7
13. Diener HC, Dichgans J, Gundalin J, Seboldt H, Huth C, Hoffmeister HE (1989) Asymptomatische Karotisstenose: Ist die operative Insultprophylaxe noch gerechtfertigt? Med Klin 84: 128–32
14. Hennerici M, Rautenberg W, Mohr S (1982) Stroke risk from symptomless extracranial artery disease. Lancet 11: 1180
15. Hennerici M, Hülsbömer HB, Hefter H, Lammerts D, Rautenberg W (1987) Natural history of asymptomatic extracranial arterial disease. Brain 110: 777–791
16. Hobson RW 2d, Towne J (1989) Carotid endarterectomy for asymptomatic carotid stenosis (editorial). Stroke 20: 575–6
17. Hobson RW 2d, Towne J (1989) The role of carotid endarterectomy in asymptomatic carotid stenosis: status of the Veterans Administration study (letter). J Vasc Surg 9: 400–1
18. Marx P (1990) Therpiekonzept bei symptomatischer Karotisstenose: Operationsindikation aus neurologischer Sicht im Vergleich zum Spontanverlauf. Langenbeck, Arch Chir Suppl I Verh Dhd Ges Forsch Chir 537–542
19. North American Symptomatic Carotid Endarterectomy Trial Collaborators (1991) Beneficial effect of carotid endarterectomy in symptomatic patients with high-grade carotid stenosis: J Med 7

20. Norris JW, Zhu CZ, Bornstein NM, Chambers BR (1991) Vascular risks of asymptomatic carotid stenosis. Stroke 22: 1485–90
21. Roederer GO, Langlois YE, Jäger KA, Primozich JF, Beach KW, Philips DJ, Strandness E (1984) The natural history of carotid arterial disease in asymptomatic patients with cervical bruits. Stroke 15: 605–613
22. Vollmar J (1982) Rekonstruktive Chirurgie der Arterien. Georg Thieme, Stuttgart New York
23. Widder B (1987) Transkranielle Doppler-Sonographie bei zerebrovaskulären Erkrankungen. Springer, Berlin Heidelberg New York Tokyo
24. Widder B, Kornhuber HH (1987) Wann ist die Carotisoperation noch indiziert? Dtsch med Wschr 112: 405–407
25. White DN, Curry GR (1977) Colour coded differential Doppler ultrasonic scanning system for the carotid bifurcation. Experta Medica Amsterdam/Oxford
26. Zhu CZ, Norris JW (1991) A therapeutic window for carotid endarterectomy in patients with asymptomatic carotid stenosis. Ca J Surg 34: 437–40

Author's address:
Dr. med. K. Balzer
Leit. Arzt der Abt. Gefäßchirurgie
Evangelisches Krankenhaus
Wertgasse 30
D-45468 Mülheim/R., Germany

Lesions of the aortic arch branches: long term results after surgical procedures

W. Hepp, A. Coutelle, W. Otto

Orthopedic University Hospital and Outpatients Clinic, Free University Berlin, Department of Vasular Surgery

Abstract

From 1971 to 1991, 76 patients were operated on for lesions of aortic arch branches (83 surgical procedures). Surgical therapy and long term results will be presented.

In 80.7 % of the procedures, extrathoracic surgical methods were performed, overwhelming as carotid-subclavian bypasses using knitted dacron grafts (6 mm and 8 mm, respectively). A transthoracic approach was used 19.3 % of the time. No patients died after operation and no ischemic neurological deficits occured. The cumulative survival rate was 92.81 % after three years and 84.16 % after seven. No failure occured within the first 30 days after operation. The early graft patency (up to one year) was 96.1 % and the late patency rate ranged 91.8 % (mean follow up of 83.2 months). In the subgroup with the transthoracic approach, the cumulative patency was 100 % after five years and ten years, respectively.

A total of 91.6 % of the patients have been symptom-free and 8.4 % improved.

The results verify that surgical procedures due to lesions of the aortic arch branches show very good long term patency results.

Introduction

In contrast to stenoses of the internal carotid artery, lesions of the aortic arch branches rarely require surgical treatment (1, 3, 4, 9, 10, 12, 13).

Long-term results of such operations have been seldom reported (8, 10, 12). Therefore, the long-term results over a 20 year time period of our own group shall be presented here.

Patients and treatment

From January 1971 through June 1991, 83 operations due to occlusive disease of the aortic arch branches were performed on a total of 76 patients. The average age was 56.4 years and the ratio male:female was 1.5:1.0.

Symptoms

In a total of 69.9 %, combined symptoms of vertebrobasilar and brachial insufficiency were dominant, only 1.2 % displayed vertebrobasilar insufficiency, and in 15.7 % brachial insufficiency was found. Remarkably, there were 10.8 % with carotid insufficiency. 2.4 % of the patients were asymptomatic; both of them needed a vascular access for hemodialysis treatment (Table 1). The involved arteries are listed in Table 2.

Surgical procedures

The surgical methods described here represent about 8 % of the total number of operations performed in the supraaortic arterial region, which supplies the brain. Carotid subclavian bypass preponderated with 52.8 % (Table 3).

Results

Neither perioperative ischemic deficit nor postoperative mortality occured in any of the patients. Only once did peripheral lesion of the hypoglossal nerve take place, subsequent

Table 1. Preoperative symptoms

	No.	%
• asymptomatic	2	2.4
• combined symptomatic	58	69.9
• vertebrobasilar insuff.	1	1.2
• brachial insufficiency	13	15.7
• carotid insufficiency	9	10.8
total	83	

Table 2. Involved arteries

involved arteries		n	%
• subclavian a.		61	70.1
– left	51		
– right	10		
• common carotid a.		12	13.8
– left	8		
– right	4		
• brachiocephalic trunc		14	16.1
total		87	

to the carotid subclavian bypass with simultaneous ipsilateral carotid endarterectomy in 1972. This was followed by complete remission of the nerval damage. The perioperative complications are registered in Table 4.

Early results (within 12 months after operation)

The surgical unrelated mortality rate registered 4.1 %, i.e., three patients out of a total of 73. The bypass patency measured 97.2 %.

Long-term results (more than 12 months)

The first time we had reported about these operations (end point 1987) in 1991 51 of 62, or 82.61 %, of the patients were living at the end of this time period. This represents a cumulative survival rate of 50.99 %, the rate after five years was 88.86 %, and after 10 years it totaled 59.49 %.

Now in 1992 49 operations, performed on 44 patients, could be checked (Table 5). 26 patients with 28 operations died in the mean time (unrelated to the surgical procedures) and six patients could not be located.

Symptom-free were 45 operations, three had improved and one had not improved (Table 6). Dopplersonographic examinations were be performed on 35 reconstructive operations (Table 7).

Table 3. Surgical procedures

	No.	%
• endarterectomy	2	2.4
• endarterectomy + patch	6	7.2
• resection + end-to-end-sut.	2	2.4
• subclavian transposition	8	9.6
• Y-graft/thoracic	5	6.0
• bypass graft	60	72.3
– carotid subclav. bypass 44		
total	83	

Table 4. Perioperative complications

	No.	%
• central neurologic deficit	1	1.2
• peripheral nerve lesion	3	3.6
• afterbleeding	6	7.2
• wound infection stage I	4	4.8
• pulmonic	5	6.0
• cardiac	1	1.2

Postoperative failure

No patient showed an immediate graft failure (within 48 hours after operation). Three patients (3.6 %) sustained early occlusion (within 48 hours until 12 months after operation). Late occlusion could be observed in three of the 49 checked up on operations (Table 8).

Table 5. No. of checked up patients

Long-term follow up 1992
• 44 pat./49 op. checked up • 26 pat./28 op. died • 6 pat./ 6 op. not located

Table 6. Clinical long-term results

Long-term check up 1992 (n = 49)	
– follow up: 8 months – 21 years (~ 83.2 months)	
• inconspicuous	45
• improved	3
• not improved	1

Table 7. Postoperative long-term dopplersonographic findings

Long-term check up 1992 (No. = 35) (dopplersonographic examination)	
• inconspicuous	30
• incomplete steal	1
• complete steal	1
• anastomotic turbulences	2
• impossible to judge	1

Table 8. Postoperative graft failure

	No.	%
• immediate occlusion	0	0.0
• early occlusion	3	3.9
• late occlusion	3/49	8.2

Discussion

Due to the polymorbidity prevalent among this group of patients, the extrathoracic, extra-anatomical surgical measures offered by carotid subclavian bypass surgery and its modifications haven been increasingly accepted since this procedure was first introduced by Barner and Dietrich in 1967 (1, 6). Since 1973, the competitive method of carotid subclavian transposition has also been established (7, 8, 11). The autologous vein has proven to be unsuitable in carotid subclavian bypass surgery, making the use of synthetic material unavoidable. The advantage of transposition lies in the fact that no interposition, and consequently no plastic material, is required here, but only one anastomosis, the operation of which is not problematic in slender patients (11). For these reasons, we also added transposition to our repertoire and have been well satisfied with the results. However, we have used this method only eight times. With patients who are adipose, short-necked, and exhibit a deep situs, however, topographic considerations have prevented us from attempting this procedure. In these cases, we have chosen to remain with the bypass method, which we find to be less time-consuming and traumatizing for this group of patients, and which, in our opinion, functions in an equally trouble-free manner (12). Further arguments advanced against the extrathoracic bypass procedures pertain to postoperative hemodynamic disturbances (11). These include claims of tubulences at the distal anastomosis, undulating blood flow of the vertebral artery, and continued or new appearance of flow inversion in this artery. But hemodynamic problems following transposition have been also reported (2). These hemodynamic consequences have been less than satisfactory, as confirmed by postoperative ultrasonography. The earlier reported long-term control examinations of our own group of patients after carotid subclavian bypass surgery have shown 84.38 % of the patients to have inconspicuous hemodynamic relations and 93.75 % to have orthograde vertebral flow without clinical symptoms (9). A disturbance in hemodynamics existed only in the three patients having had bypass failures. Long-term control examinations have shown the 6 mm caliber graft, which had three failures, to be unsuitable. The results presented here document carotid subclavian bypass surgery using dacron grafts as a method which produces little stress and exhibits an extremely low surgical mortality rate. Using 8 mm grafts, functional findings have shown excellent long-term results, registering no failures during a 20-year period time with a mean observation interval of eight years.

The results verify that surgical procedures due to lesions of the aortic arch branches, and hereby the carotid subclavian bypass particularily, show very good long term patency results.

References

1. Barner HB, Rittenhouse EA, Willman VL (1968) Carotid subclavian bypass for "subclavian steal syndrome". J Thorac Cardiovasc Surg 55: 773–782
2. Cormier JM, Laurian C, Franceschi C, Luizy F (1985) Réimplantation de la sous-clavière dans la carotide primitive. La Presse Médicale 14: 1512–1517
3. Crawford ES, DeBakey ME, Morris GC, Howell JF (1969) Surgical treatment of the occlusion of innominate, common carotid and subclavian arteries: A ten years' experience. Surgery 65: 17–31
4. DeBakey ME, Crawford ES, Cooley DA, Morris JC, Garrett HE, Fields WS (1965) Cerebral arterial insufficiency: one to eleven years following arterial reconstruction operation. Ann Surg 161: 921–930

5. DeJonge K, Hepp W, Haase T, Hampl H (1986) Seltene Indikation zur Rekonstruktion einer zentralen Arteria sublavia-Stenose. In: Häring R, Berichtsband 5. Gemeinsame Jahrestagung der Angiologischen Gesellschaften der Bundesrepublik Deutschland, Österreichs und der Schweiz, Berlin 1985. Demeter, Gräfelfing, pp 524–525

6. Dietrich EB, Garrett HE, Ameriso J, Crawford ES, El-Bavar M, DeBakey ME (1967) Occlusive disease of the common carotid and subclavian arteries treated by carotid-subclavian bypass. Analysis of 125 cases. Am J Surg 114: 800–807

7. Edwards WH, Mulherin JL Jr (1984) The surgical reconstruction of the proximal subclavian and vertebral artery. In: Berguer R, Bauer RB (eds): Vertebrobasilar Arterial Occlusive Disease. Raven Press, New York, pp 241–255

8. Edwards WH Jr, Tapper SS, Edwards WH Sr, Mulherin JH, Martin RS III, Jenkins JM (1994) Subclavian revascularisation: A Quarter Century Experience. Ann Surg 219: 673–678

9. Hepp W, Dieruff M, Otto W (1991) Strombahnblockaden an den Aortenbogenästen: Chirurgische Behandlung und Langzeitergebnisse. Zbl Chirurgie 116: 613–622

10. Salam TA, Lumbsden AB, Smith RB III (1994) Subclavian artery revascularisation: A decade of experience with extrathoracic bypass procedures. J Surg Res 56: 387–392

11. Sandmann W, Kniemeyer HW, Jaeschock R, Hennerici M, Aulich A (1987) The role of carotid-subclavian transposition in surgery for supraaortic occlusive disease. J Vasc Surg 5: 53–58

12. Vitti MJ, Thompson BW, Read RC, Gagne PJ, Barone GW, Barnes RW, Eidt JF (1994) Carotid-Subclavian Bypass: A twenty-two-year experience. J Vasc Surg 20: 411–418

13. Vollmar JF (1996) Rekonstruktive Chirurgie der Arterien. 4. edition Thieme, Stuttgart New York

Author's address:
Prof. Dr. med. W. Hepp
St. Josef-Krankenhaus
Department of Vascular Surgery
Robert-Koch-Straße 16
42781 Haan, Germany

Operative results after reconstruction of extracranial carotid artery aneurysms (ECAA)

K. Ktenidis, Ch. Winkler, K. Simons, S. Horsch

Department of Vascular Surgery, Krankenhaus Porz am Rhein, University of Cologne Teaching Hospital, Cologne

Introduction

Extracranial carotid aneurysm are uncommon, but their clinical significance has long been recognized. Indeed, surgical treatment like proximal ligation was first employed successfully in 1808 (2). In 1952 Dimtza introduced the reconstructive operation, but the first successful reconstruction (aneurysm resection with end-to-end anastomosis) was carried out by Shea in 1955 (2, 3, 4).

Schechter found reports of a total of only 853 carotid artery aneurysms in the literature up to 1977 (8). McCollum et al. reported only 37 carotid aneurysms out of a total of 8500 surgically treated aneurysms in the 20 years up to 1977 (5). Welling et al. reported 41 carotid aneurysms from a total of 1118 peripheral aneurysms evaluated during 30-year period (10). Busuttil et al. found that while 500 patient with occlusive carotid disease had been dealt with over a 24-year period, only 19 carotid aneurysms were treated in the same period (1). The total incidence of extracranial carotid artery aneurysm is relative small. The incindence of this aneurysm type compared to the other peripheral aneurysms lay between 0.4 and 3.7 % (1, 4–10).

Many causes of the carotid aneurysms have been discribed, but the most important are atherosclerosis and trauma. The atherosclerotic aneurysm usually occurs in elderly and hypertensive patients. This aneurysm type is frequently associated with other atherosclerotic arterial disease and is preferably localized in the region of bifurcation (4, 6, 9). In most cases, the diagnosis can be made clinically without difficulty. However, enlarged lymph nodes, cervical cysts, carotid body tumors, and elongated or kinked carotid arteries may occassionally be confused. Here, it may only be possible to prove the diagnosis with arteriography or ultrasound examination. Apart from the patient's history and clinical examination, ultrasound scanning angiography is the essential investigative method, when surgical reconstruction is planned. Additionally, the computertomography (cerebral CT, Angio-CT) is necessary preoperatively. The complete diagnostic management contains neurological and otorhinolaryngological examination before and after the operation (4, 6, 9).

Method, material and results

Nowdays, the aneurysm resection and graft interposition is the treatment of choice. The resection and patch angioplasty are possible in cases of small saccular aneurysms. The simple ligation of the carotid artery is from historic significance (4, 6, 9).

The operative technique is standardized and the important surgical steps are as follows: After the cervical skin incision along the anterior border of the sternocleidomastoid muscle, electrosurgical division of the subcutis and platysma is performed. This is followed by incision of the cervical superficial fascia, mobilization of the strernocleidomastoid muscle, opening of the carotid sheath, division and ligation of the transverse facial vein, lateral preparation of the cervical lymph node, high dissection of internal carotid artery (in the level of the digastricus muscle), good care of hypoglusus nerve and ansa hypoglosi, and systemic heparinization (100 units per kilogram). In order to avoid cerebral embolisation, the internal carotid artery is clamped cranial to aneurysm with recording of somatosensory evoked potentials or other monitoring method. (Alternative procedure: dissecting und clamping of common carotid artery proximal to the aneurysm after systemic heparinization and under cerebral monitoring). Next is complete dissection of the carotid arteries and aneurysm, and with inconspicuousness of cerebral monitoring complete clamping of the carotid arteries. Reconstruction without intraluminal shunt includes: segmental resection and graft interposition as therapy of choice, resection and patchplasty (small saccular aneurysms), or in extreme situations proximal and distal ligation of carotid artery (6, 9).

From January 1986 to November 1996, 25 patients with a total of 29 carotid aneurysm were treated. There were 20 men and 5 women with the mean age of 56.7 years (range: 5–87). Overall, 3747 operations of the internal carotid artery were performed during the same period, the incidence of these aneurysms, thus, being 0.8 per cent. In 20 cases, we were dealing with true aneurysms, whereas the other eight cases were postreconstructive pseudoaneurysms. One false carotid aneurysm resulted after a knife-injury and was observed in a five-year old child. Apart from eight asymptomatic cases, 17 patients showed neurological deficits. In 7 cases patients complained of symptoms of local displacement and a palpable mass.

No patient died postoperatively (30-day mortality). We did not obeserved any stroke event (30-day morbidity). Two patients suffered transitoric ischemic attack (TIA). In 13.7 % we registered temporary cranial nerve lesions (3 reccurens nerve and 1 hypoglossal nerve, 1 Horner syndrome). In two cases we registered graft (ePTFE) occlusion without neurology.

Discussion

The most common causes for extracranial carotid artery aneurysm are atherosclerosis and trauma. The postreconstructive carotid aneurysm is more and more frequent in our days for a special type of traumatic aneurysm. The incidence of this aneurysm is low (0.4 to 3.7 %), but its significance is undisputed because of the high rate of possible severe complications (1, 4–10).

The sufficient therapy is based on perfect perioperative management. The diagnosis of a carotid aneurysm automatically necessitates a surgical approach due to the risk of thromboembolic complications provoking neurological deficits, rupture, and local displacement (4, 6). Our results demonstrate no mortality and morbitity with regard to permanent neurological deficits (0 %). As prosthesis we have used only a good saphenous vein or ePTFE graft (4, 6, 7, 9, 10).

In conclusion, any palpable cervical tumor must be considered to be a carotid aneurysm. The coincidental occurence of neurological symptoms calls for immediate diagnosis and therapy because of the seriousness of possible complications.

References

1. Busuttil RW, Davidson RK, Foley KT, Livesay JT, Barker WF (1980) Selective management of extracranial carotid arterial aneurysms. Am J Surg 140: 85
2. Cooper A (1936) Account of the first successful operation performed on the common carotid artery for aneurysm in the year of 1808 with post mortem examination in the year 1821. Guy's Hosp Reo 1: 53
3. Dimtza A (1956) Aneurysms of the carotid arteries. report of two cases. Angiology 7: 218
4. Gillespie JA (1987) Extracranial carotis artery aneurysms In: Vascular Surgery – Principles and Practice. S. E. Wilson, F. J. Veith, R. W. Hobson, R. A. Williams. McGraw-Hill. Inc.
5. McCollum CH, Wheeler WG, Noon GP, DeBakey ME (1979) Aneurysms of the extracranial carotid artery. twenty-one years experience. Am J Surg 137: 196
6. Raithel D (1989) Arterielle Aneurysmen der extracraniellen supraaortalen Äste. In: Gefäßchirurgie. G. Heberer, RJAM van Dongen. Springer-Verlag, Berlin
7. Sahlman A, Salo J, Kostiainen S, Lahti P, Aarnio P, Harjula A (1991) Extracranial carotid aneurysm. Vasa 20: 369–373
8. Schlechter DC (1979) Cervical carotid aneurysms. NY State J Med 79: 892
9. Vollmar J (1995) Rekonstruktive Chirurgie der Arterien. Thieme-Verlag, Stuttgart
10. Welling RE, Taha A, Goel T, Cranley J, Krause R, Hafner C, Tew J (1983) Extracranial carotid artery aneurysms. Surgery 93: 319

Author's address:
Kiriakos Ktenidis, MD
Krankenhaus Porz am Rhein,
Teach.-Hospital of Univ. of Cologne
Department of General and Vascular Surgery
Urbacher Weg 19
51149 Köln, Germany

Carotid surgery before vertebral artery reconstruction: long-term results (1989–1994)

J. Marsch, P. Gierloff, M. Zaiac, I. Flessenkaemper, T. Gramsdorff

Surgical Dept., Rittberg-Krankenhaus, Berlin, Germany

Dear Chairmen, Ladies and Gentlemen,

our study is pointing out the importance of carotid surgery for patients suffering from non-hemispheric symptoms, formerly described as vertebro-basilar symptoms. According to the World Health Organisation, cerebrovascular disease is classified into four stages. Of special interest are the asymptomatic stage I and stage II, which includes the monocular blindness, transitory ischaemic attack and minor stroke. European (ECST) and American (NASCET) studies proved the carotid stenosis > 70 % to be an indication for carotid endarterectomy. Trials are still in progress to assess the following pathologies of carotid artery as indication for surgery: stenosis > 90 %; stenosis > 70 %; progressive stenosis; stenosis and/or ulceration with undetected stroke; stenosis > 70 % with non-hemispheric symptoms.

During the years 1989 to 1994 we did 427 reconstructions of supraaortic branches in total. Of these 355 carotid endarterectomies were performed. The rate of morbidity following operation was 2.6 % and one patient died 15 days after operation from heart attack. We operated on 122 patients for asymptomatic cerebrovascular disease, according to WHO stage I. This group consists of 58 patients being operated prior to bypass-surgery as coronary heart and peripheral vascular disease. In terms of staging these really were asymptomatic, whereas the remainder of the group had symptoms described as non-hemispheric or vertebro-basilar.

On special investigation of a patient's history and/or carotid bruits we first do a duplex-scan. At the same time we have a cardiologist and an ENT-specialist examining the patient. If the duplex-scan shows pathology, intra-arterial arch digital subtraction angiography and CCT or NMR is done. In the planning of surgery on the Art. carotis or vertebralis a neurologist is involved. In total 136 patients were operated on supraaortic branches for vertebral insufficiency; 56 patients had vertebral and 16 had surgery on the Art. subclavia. The largest group of 64 patients underwent carotid endarterectomy. Our follow-up study is concentrating on these carotid patients. The follow-up date was 1 to 6 years (mean, 3.7 years) after surgery had been performed, 20 % of whom have had previous surgery on contralateral Art. carotis interna. The patients were 28 to 85 years old (mean, 68.3 years). The females dominated the males in 71 to 29 %; an interesting rate knowing that in studies for stage II carotid-surgery the males dominate.

The leading symptoms were vertigo (73 % of cases), headache (35 %), disturbance of coordination (25 %) and visual disturbances (26 %) other than monocular blindness. Others were transitory ischaemic attack (TIA) or minor stroke more than 6 months previously (19 %), psychic disorders (19 %) ranging from recent difficulties in concentrating to a depressive syndrome. Patients complained of par- and dysaethesia in the face, limbs or trunk (13 %) and audial disturbances, i.e. tinnitus (7 %). Undetected stroke was found in 10 % of cases.

Postoperatively the majority of patients felt free of any symptoms or improved:

	Free of symptoms (%)	Improved (%)	Unchanged (%)
Vertigo	60	36	4
Headache	48	35	17
Disturbances of coordination	38	28	34
Visual disturbances	60	28	12
Results of angiography of all patients operated for vertebral insufficiency (n = 136)			
Unilateral vertebral lesion	7 %		
Unilateral vertebral lesion and carotid insufficiency	28 %		
Bilateral vertebral lesion	10 %		
Bilateral vertebral lesion and carotid insufficiency	55 %		
Results of angiography of all patients operated on Art. carotis for vertebral insufficiency (n = 64)			
Unilateral carotid lesion	16 %		
Unilateral carotid lesion and vertebral insufficiency	18 %		
Bilateral carotid lesion	28 %		
Bilateral carotid lesion and vertebral insufficiency	38 %		

The results of angiography show that about 40 % of patients suffering from vertebral insufficiency only show uni- or bilateral carotid lesion but not a vertebral one. Discussing the importance of carotid surgery for vertebral insufficiency, the problems of vertebral surgery have to be mentioned. In general vertebral reconstruction relies on greater skill of the surgeon. The anatomy is more difficult than in carotid surgery. The location of the Art. vertebralis, its delicate wall, surroundings veins and nerves add to the difficulties. Vertebral surgery needs a well-documented circle of Willis, possibly with selective angiogram. Prolonged operation time and higher morbidity add to the problems.

In conclusion carotid surgery is proved for stage II. Trials such as ACAS[1] and ACST[2] are in progress for stage I; several indications are still being discussed. Of our patients 30 % show clinical signs of vertebral insufficiency. Angiograms show about 70 % of combined carotid and vertebral lesions and 20 % of carotid lesions only; in these cases there is an indication for carotid reconstruction prior to operation on the vertebral artery. In half of the cases carotid endarterectomy was done, the other half had vertebral or subclavian reconstruction. We reviewed our carotid patients during the period of 1 to 5 years after operation; 80 % felt improved, of whom 60 % were free of symptoms. Only 10 % had to undergo vertebralis reconstruction as well. Carotid surgery has a high therapeutic benefit additional to its prophylactic value to protect from stroke.

[1] Asymptomatic Carotid Atherscleroris Study (USA)
[2] Asymptomatic Carotid Surgery Trial (UK + Europ)

Author's address:
J. Marsch, M.D.
Department of Vascular Surgery
German Red Cross Hospital
Mark Brandenburg
Drontheimer Straße 39–40
13359 Berlin, Germany

Ex vivo quantification of carotid stenoses: evaluation of eversion endarterectomy specimen

H.-H. Eckstein[1], H. Schumacher[1], K. Post[2], E. Hoffmann[1], W. Gross[3], J.-R. Allenberg[1]

1 Department of Surgery (Prof. Dr. Ch. Herfarth),
   Division of Vascular Surgery (Prof. Dr. J. R. Allenberg), University of Heidelberg
2 Department of Radiodiagnostics (Prof. Dr. G. W. Kauffmann), University of Heidelberg
3 Department of Experimental Surgery (Prof. Dr. M. Gebhardt), University of Heidelberg

Introduction

Since being presented the results of the two major multicenter trials ECST (European Carotid Surgery Trial) and NASCET (North American Symptomatic Carotid Surgery Trial), it is very decisive to precisely evaluate the degree of symptomatic carotid artery stenosis prior to the procedure with regard to the specific therapeutic management decision: carotid endarterectomy in angiographically verified stenosis >70 % or standard medical treatment with antiplatelet agents, primarily aspirin, in mild or moderate stenosis (10, 20). Due to different angiographic measurement formula, the results of both studies are not directly comparable with each other: while in the ECST trial the residual lumina were compared with the estimated original lumina at the site of the stenosis ("local degree of stenosis"), the so-called distal degree of stenosis was calculated by charging the ratio between the residual lumina and the diameter of the intact distal internal carotid artery. These different measurements are the reason, that the local degree of a 82 % stenosis (ECST criteria) corresponds with the distal degree of a 70 % stenosis (NASCET criteria); to a local degree of a 50 % stenosis no distal degree of stenosis can be calculated (0 %).

The valence of both Doppler and/or Duplex ultrasound as a non-invasive screening procedure and of additional diagnostic techniques of higher-grade carotid stenoses is not yet clearly defined. While there is a high conformity to the angiography documented by very skilled investigators in several studies, the NASCET-investigators found an overestimation of the angiographically obtained degree of stenosis in 21 % and an underestimation in 33 % (2, 14, 28). "Weak points" of Doppler/Duplex ultrasound are among others the investigator dependence, the result transfer with different Duplex equipment, and the difficulties in the differentiation between pseudo-occlusion and complete occlusion of the internal carotid artery.

Reviewing the literature, it is amazing that there are only a few, sometimes critically rated validating studies to evaluate the preoperative diagnostic imaging data by means of determining the extent of reduction in cross-section respectively in plane at the endarterectomy specimen (6, 11, 23, 25, 27, 29). Two actual specimen investigations point out that the real degree of stenosis might also be underestimated – certainly in a small case number – in the selective angiography as the present gold standard (1, 21).

Carotid eversion endarterectomy makes it possible to often obtain completely intact stenosis cylinders not being changed or destroyed through any arterectomy in the area of the maximum stenosis (9, 15). In our own pilot study we were able to demonstrate that such carotid eversion cylinders are suitable for ex vivo evaluation of the degree of carotid artery stenosis directly at the site of the speciman (8). In collaboration with the Department of Experimental Surgery, we performed a comparison study between the local and distal degree of stenosis at the carotid eversion cylinder (reduction in diameter and plane).

Material and methods

Fifty-four carotid eversion cylinders could be evaluated in the period March 1994 to February 1995, being preserved in the course of carotid eversion endarterectomy. Intra-operatively the caliber of the distal internal carotid artery prior to endarterectomy were calculated using a micrometer. Intraarterial digital subtraction angiography (aortic arch angiography n = 27, selective angiography n = 27) was made 2 – 30 days preoperatively: anterior-posterior (ap), right (RAO) and left anterior oblique (LAO) projections were simultaneously performed, the amount of contrast medium was 40 ml for selective technique applied manually, and 100 ml for the general angiography injected mechanically; the contrast medium (Solutrast, BYK Gulden, Konstanz, Germany) was diluted in a 1:3 ratio with common salt solution, the flow rate was 10 – 15 ml/s. Not knowing the intra-operative situation, the local and distal degrees of stenosis were evaluated according to the ECST and NASCET criteria (Fig. 1).

The quantification of carotid stenosis in the eversion specimen was made after formalin fixation using the polymer methylmethacrylate (Palavit M, Heraeus Kulzer GmbH, Wehr-heim, Germany) typically used in dentistry. The fluid acrylate was injected under pressure via a knob probe into the eversion cylinders and within a few minutes it polymerized. There was a local dissection in 12 cases (partially due to missing lumina); these specimens were excluded from further investigation. After a longitudinal incision of the atherosclerotic cylinder, the polymerized cast was removed and the smallest diameter at the site of the maximum stenosis was determined using a micrometer. Calculating the proportion between smallest diameter of stenosis and local vessel diameter (at the eversion cylinder), the local degree of stenosis was determined at the specimen. For evaluation of the distal degree of stenosis at the specimen, the coefficient of stenosis obtained from the acrylate cast was compared with the intraoperatively measured diameter of the distal internal carotid artery in consideration of wall thickness of 1 mm. For calculating the reduction in plane, the acrylate cast cylinder was transversely divided at the maximum site of stenosis and an ink mark was made from the "stenosis plane". This ink mark was planimetrically video-assisted measured using a special software ("Capimage", Steinzl, Heidelberg). The cross-section planes from the original internal carotid artery at the site of the stenosis and the distal internal carotid artery were calculated with the help of the formula $\pi x r^2$. In the same mode as for the linear local and distal degree of stenosis, the local and distal planar degree of stenosis were also calculated.

Statistical analysis was performed by means of the non-parametric Wilcoxon matched pairs test or the paired Students t-test. A p-value < 0.05 was considered to be statistically significant. All the calculations were separately performed both for selective and non-selective (aortic arch) angiography.

Results

We were able to investigate 54 carotid eversion cylinders. The difference found between the local and distal degree of stenosis was about 8 %, both in angiography (non-selective and selective angiography) and at the specimen (diameter and plane) (Tables 1, 2).

Generally, high-grade internal carotid stenosis was partially underestimated up to > 20 %. Due to minor measurement differences, there was no guiding discrimination between the evaluation of the linear local and distal degree of stenosis at the site of the specimen (reduction in diameter) in comparison with the selective carotid angiography.

On the other hand, both the local and distal degree of stenosis were significantly underestimated in the aortic arch angiography in comparison to the intraoperative specimen ($p < 0.01$ and $p < 0.05$, Tables 1, 2). Accordingly, the sensitivity of selective angiography in the evaluation of > 70 % carotid stenosis was clearly higher (100 % for linear local stenosis and 91.3 % for local distal stenosis) as the sensitivity of the aortic arch angiography (82.5 % and only 60 %) (Figs. 1 – 4). Whereas some high-grade carotid stenosis were clearly underestimated even in the selective angiography, particularly moderate carotid stenoses (60 – 80 %) were slightly overestimated in the tendency. In special cases, the real degree of stenosis was overestimated both in the selective and non-selective angiography (with the exception of the linear local degree of stenosis, positive predictive value (PPV) 100 %), resulting in a PPV of 85.7 % for the linear distal degree of stenosis in the aortic arch angiography, 92 % for the linear local degree of stenosis in the selective angiography and 95.5 % for the linear distal degree of stenosis in the selective angiography.

Table 1. Angiographic evaluation of the local degree of stenosis in comparison to the reduction in diameter and plane at the specimen (ECST-criteria, STD = standard deviation)

	Mean (%)	Median (%)	Range (%)	STD	Wilcoxon (p)
Selective angiography (n = 27)	82.9	83	67 – 92	7,4	
specimen: linear degree of stenosis (∅)	83,3	87	56 – 97	11,1	= 0.7
specimen: planar degree of stenosis	89,5	92	67 – 99	8,4	= 0.0002
Aortic arch angiography (n = 27)	77,8	80	60 – 93	8,5	
specimen: linear degree of stenosis (∅)	82,8	83	69 – 94	6,2	= 0.007
specimen: planar degree of stenosis	91,6	95	64 – 99	7,7	= 0.00006

Table 2. Angiographic evaluation of the distal degree of stenosis in comparison to the reduction in diameter and plane at the specimen (NASCET-criteria, STD = standard deviation)

	Mean (%)	Median (%)	Range (%)	STD	Wilcoxon (p)
Selective angiography (n = 27)	75,6	75	50 – 90	10,4	
specimen: linear degree of stenosis (∅)	79	80	55 – 96	11,8	= 0.25
specimen: planar degree of stenosis	82	84	63 – 97	11,4	= 0.015
Aortic arch angiography (n = 27)	70	72	47 – 92	12,5	
specimen: linear degree of stenosis (∅)	75,9	77	63 – 91	8,5	= 0.03
specimen: planar degree of stenosis	83,4	88	53 – 98	12,3	= 0.0004

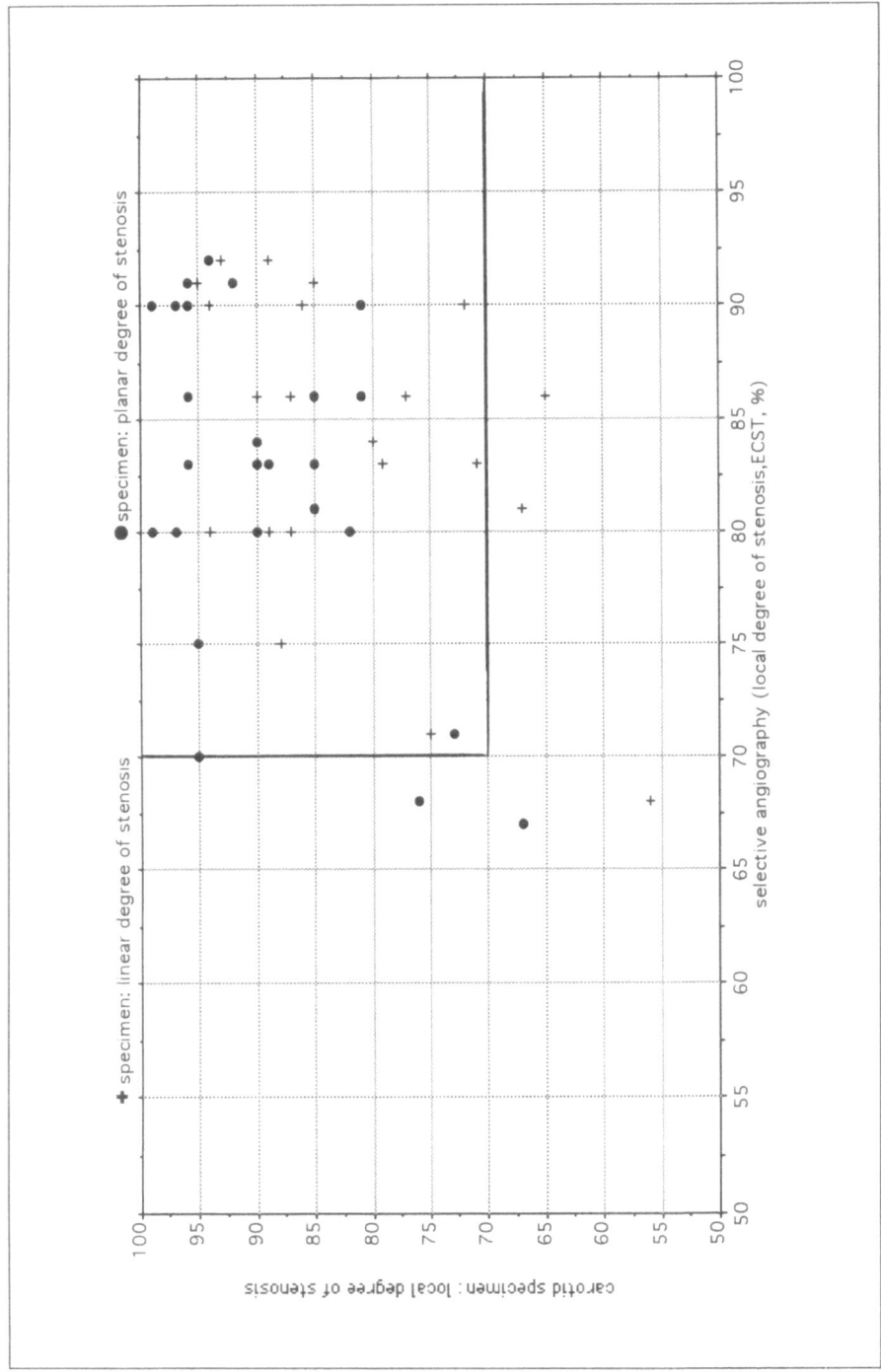

Fig. 1. Determination of the local degree of stenosis (ECST criteria) with selective angiography: comparison of the linear and planar degrees of stenosis at the carotid endarterectomy specimen.
Detection of a ≥ 70 % linear stenosis: sensitivity 100 %, positive predictive value 92 %
detection of a ≥ 70 % planar stenosis: sensitivity 96.2 %, positive predictive value 100 %

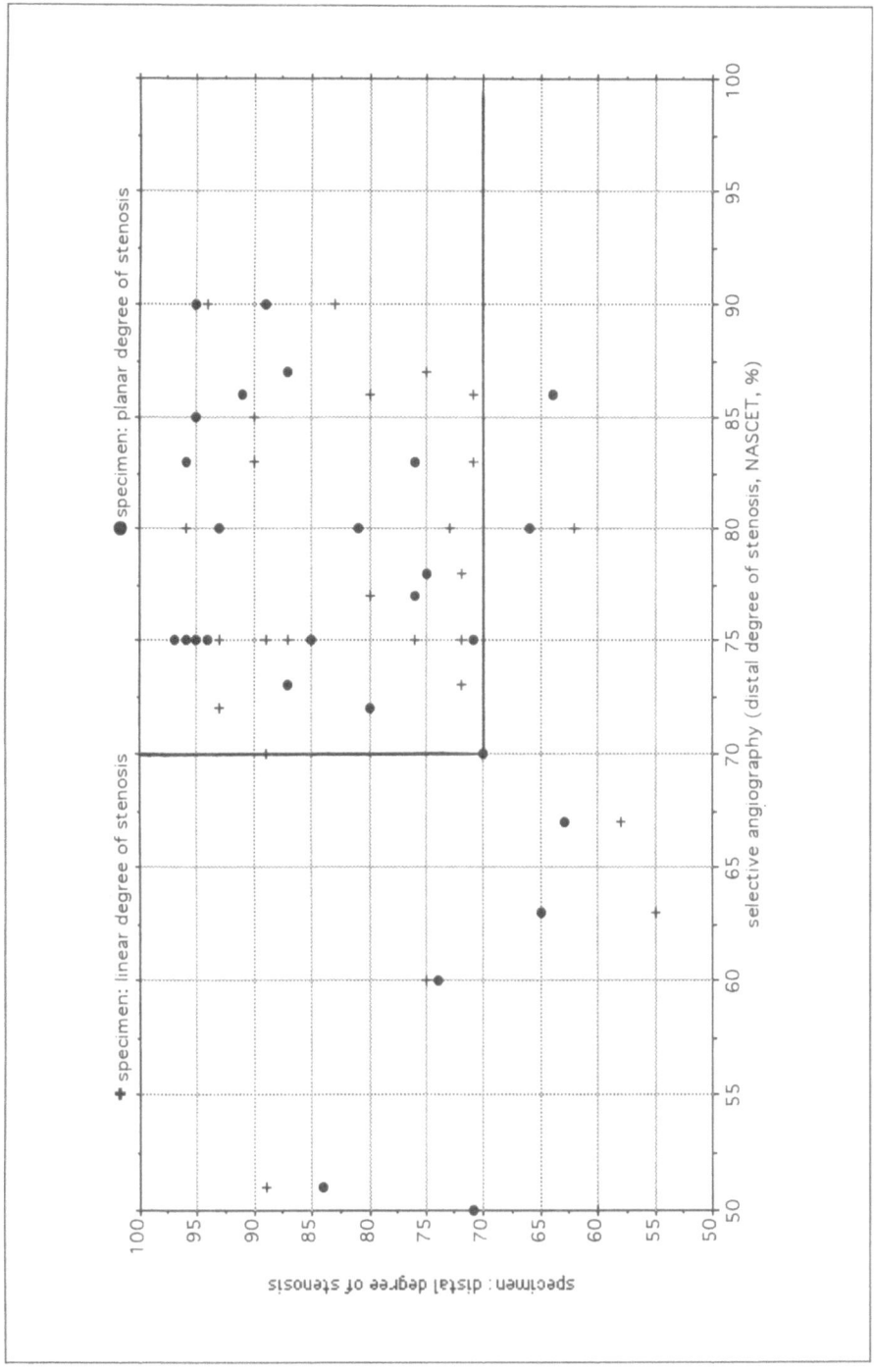

Fig. 2. Determination of the distal degree of stenosis (NASCET criteria) with selective angiography: comparison with the linear and planar degrees of stenosis at the carotid endarterectomy specimen.
Detection of a ≥ 70 % linear stenosis: sensitivity 91.3 % , positive predictive value 95.5 %
detection of a ≥ 70 % planar stenosis: sensitivity 87 % , positive predictive value 90.9 %

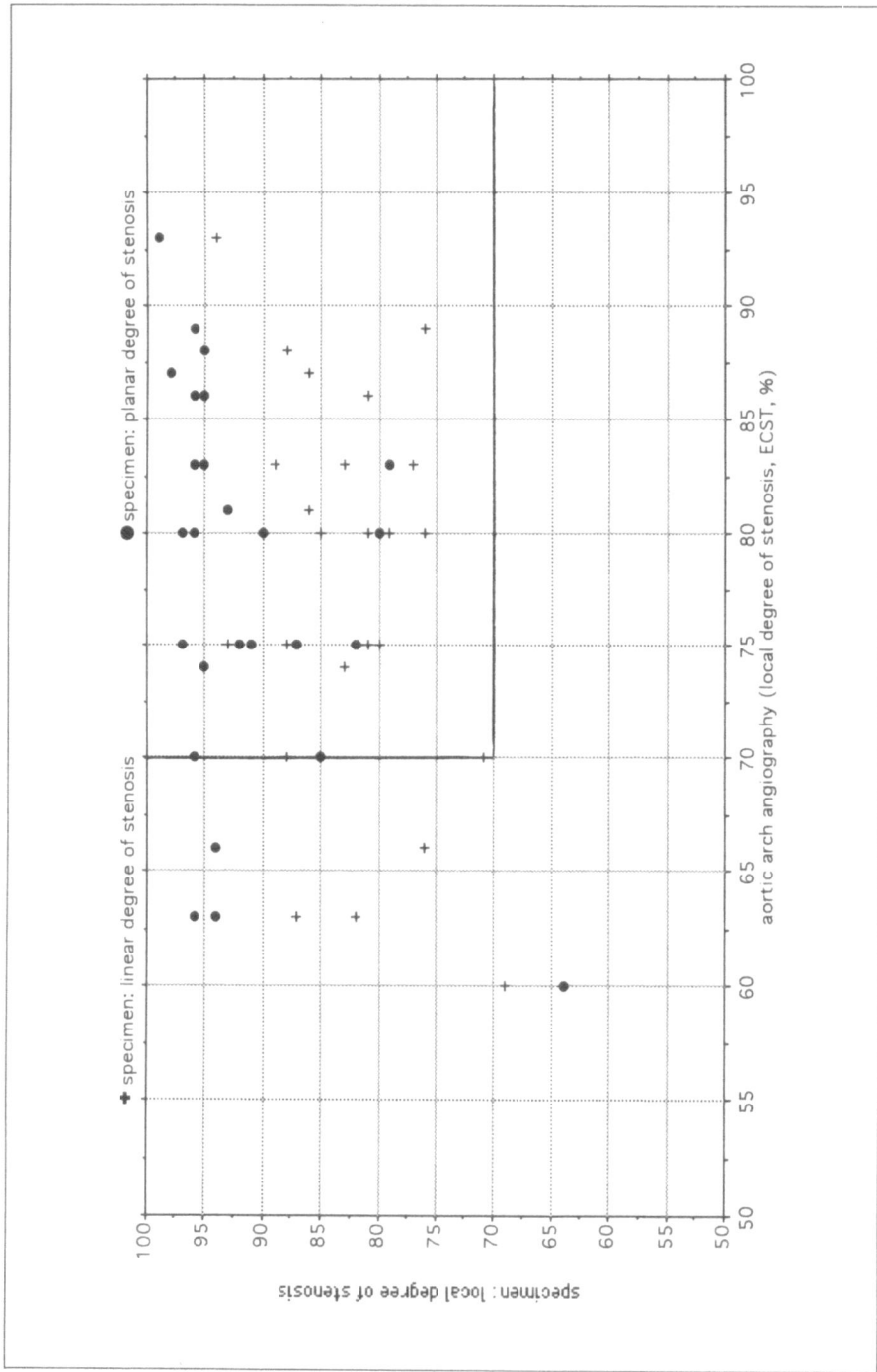

Fig. 3. Determination of the local degree of stenosis (ECST criteria) with aortic arch angiography: comparison of the linear and planar degrees of stenosis at the carotid endarterectomy specimen.
Detection of a ≥ 70 % linear stenosis: sensitivity 85.2 %, positive predictive value 100 %
detection of a ≥ 70 % planar stenosis: sensitivity 85.2 %, positive predictive value 100 %

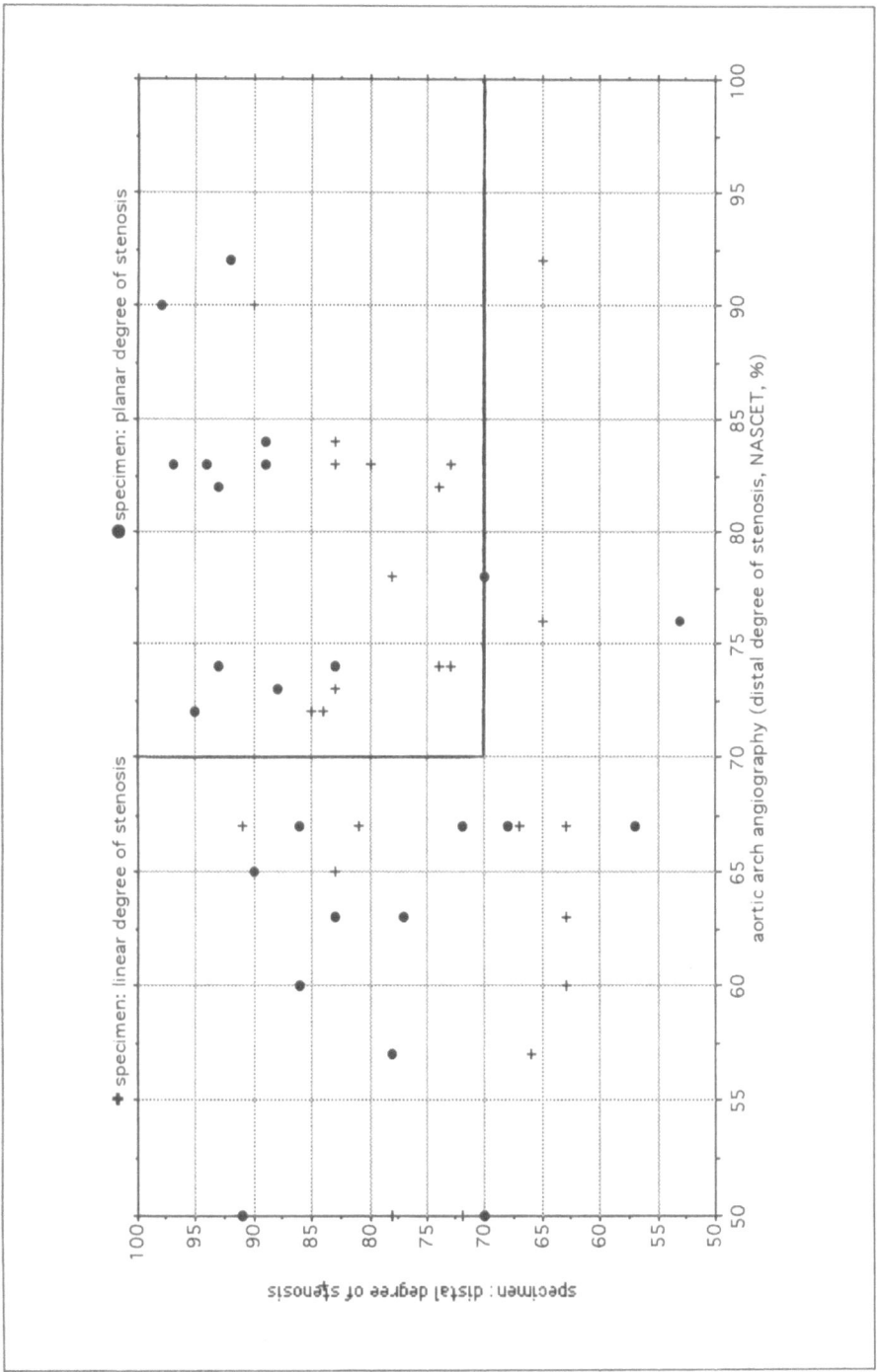

Fig. 4. Determination of the distal degree of stenosis (NASCET criteria) with aortic arch angiography: comparison with the linear and planar degrees of stenosis at the carotid endarterectomy specimen.
Detection of a ≥ 70 % linear stenosis: sensitivity 60 %, positive predictive value 85.7 %
detection of a > 70 % planar stenosis: sensitivity 56.6 %, positive predictive value 92.9 %

With a difference of 9 – 16 % (median), the planar degree of stenosis is partially under-estimated with a high significance both in the selective and aortic arch angiography (Tables 1, 2). As for the reduction of plane, the sensitivity for the selective angiography was 96.2 % (local stenosis) and 87 % (distal stenosis). The non-selective angiography with a sensitivity of only 56.6 % is not able to correctly classify the distal planar degree of stenosis for > 70 % carotid stenoses (Figs. 1 – 4).

Discussion

The extent of the stenosis of the internal carotid artery is not only the most important pre-dictor for cerebrovascular disease (stroke, transient ischemic attacks (TIA)) but also an indicator for an increased cardiovascular risk profile: Norris et al. reported for asympto-matic < 50 % carotid stenoses an annual risk rate for TIA and stroke of 1 % and 1.3 % respectively, and a risk rate for coronary artery disease (CAD) of 2.7 %. The annual CAD risk was almost 6.6 % for 50 – 75 % carotid stenoses and even 8.3 % for > 75 % stenoses (TIA and stroke risk 7.2 % and 3.3 %) (19).

Selective intraarterial angiography was the diagnostic standard so far, meanwhile there are at least four different measurement procedures for the percental quantification of carotid artery stenosis – besides the evaluation of the lumina reduction in mm: evaluation of the local and distal degree of stenosis according to the ECST or NASCET criteria, the Common Carotid method, in which the restlumen is compared to the angiographic lumen in the intact common carotid, and as the most actual suggestion according to the so-called carotid stenosis index (CSI), postulating a fixed anatomic proportion between internal carotid bulbus and common carotid artery of 1.2:1 (3, 24). All these methods have specific disadvantages: the local degree of stenosis can only be given by estimation of the original internal carotid diameter at the site of the stenosis, the distal internal carotid is sometimes poorly presented and may be "collapsed" in the case of high-grade stenosis, so that the determination of the distal degree of stenosis is also not always possible (12).

Independent of the measurement procedures, the angiographic quantification of carotid stenosis "suffers" on principle from evaluating a 3-D event by means of a linear degree of stenosis, i.e., with the help of 2-D imaging data, which is a disadvantage that cannot not be compensated by angiographic images in different projections. This is also the reason for the noticed discrepancy between the preoperative finding of a "smooth-wall" 80 % internal carotid stenosis and the intraoperative finding of a highest-grade sub-total carotid stenosis. Furthermore the linear degree of stenosis offers only inaccurate data concerning the real reduction in plane: a 50 % concentric linear stenosis corresponds arithmetically with a 75 % reduction in plane, and a 70 % linear stenosis with a 91 % planar stenosis. Duplex ultrasound, MR- and/or CT-angiography are non or less invasive diagnos-tic techniques, which were evaluated in comparison with the angiography as the gold stan-dard, although the different angiographic measurements result in totally different degrees of stenosis with different consequences for the therapeutic management (4, 18). In two actual specimen investigations with small case numbers (15 and 31 intact carotid end-arterectomy specimen) it was found out that the real degree of stenosis is sometimes underestimated also with selective angiography and that Duplex ultrasound and MR-angiography may provide more precise data (1, 21).

Reviewing the literature, there are only a small number of investigations about the exact extent of carotid stenoses using evaluation of the endarterectomy specimen. The great

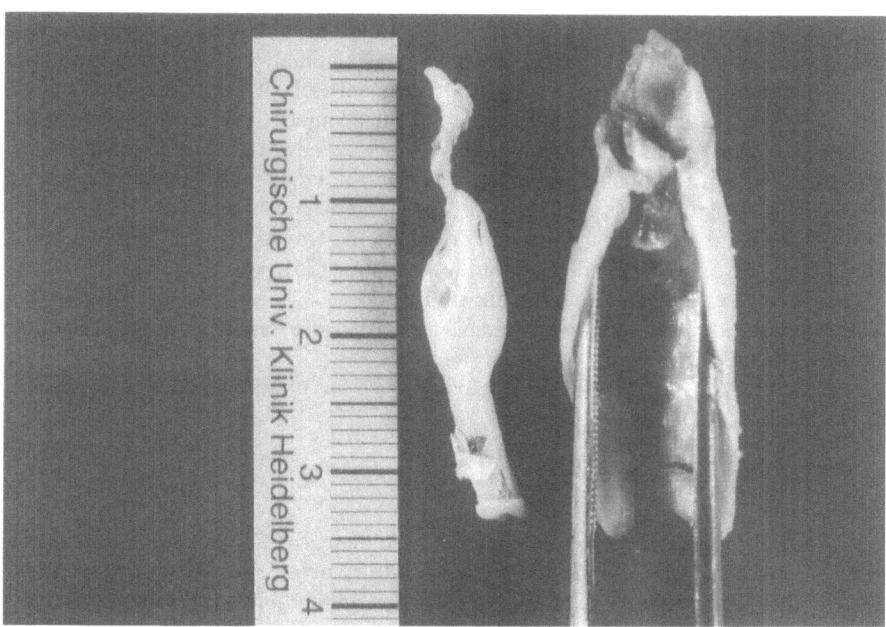

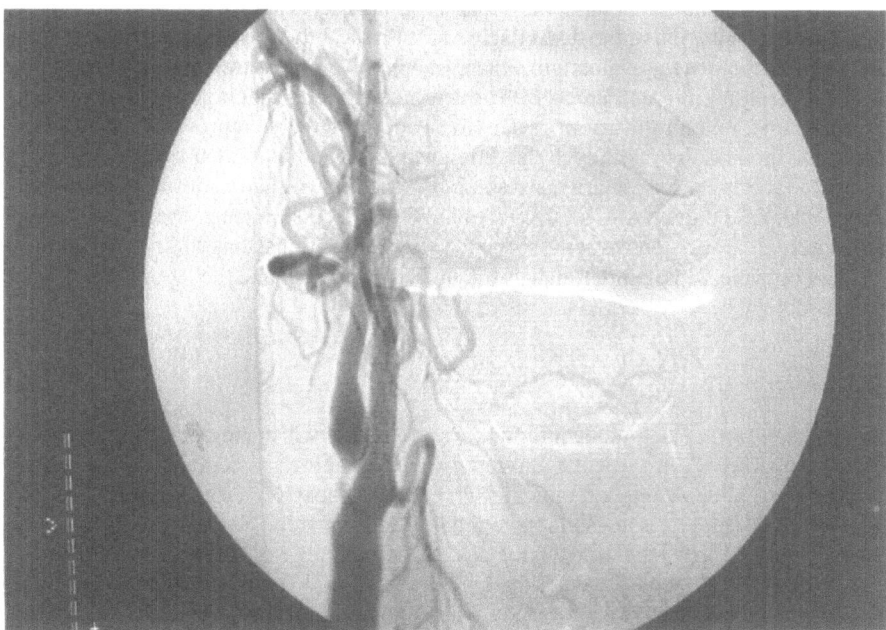

Fig. 5. Carotid eversion cylinder with the acrylate cast cylinder and the corresponding selective angiography (ECST 92 %, NASCET 80 %, specimen: local 98 %, distal 94 %, 71 yr. male TIA).

majority of these studies has to be critically judged, because the degree of stenosis was intraoperatively estimated or the preoperative imaging data resulted from intravenous digital subtraction technique (6, 11, 23, 27, 29). The main problem in methodology of these studies was the fact that it was very difficult to obtain an intact endarterectomy specimen, which can be macro- and histopathologically evaluated and are suitable to exactly determine the extent of the lumina reduction. Even in the largest evaluation study so far (B-mode ultrasound, angiography) from 5 North American centers, 53 % of all the 289 carotid specimen were fragmented or partially destroyed by the intraoperative arteriotomy, and only of limited value for the evaluation (25).

We raised two essential questions in our study:

1) Are the carotid eversion cylinders suitable for a real "gold standard" for the evaluation of the linear and planar degree of carotid stenoses?

2) What about the reliability of the angiography as the presently accepted diagnostic "gold standard"?

ad 1

The carotid eversion endarterectomy enables us in many cases to obtain intact stenosis cylinders, which are not destroyed at the stenosis site by any arteriotomy, i.e., the stenosis will be obtained like "in situ". Such eversion cylinders are suitable in particular to evaluate the degree of stenosis ex vivo. According to the literature, the fixation with formalin does not lead to any relevant shrinkage of the eversion specimen (13). The determination of the local degree of stenosis is easily possible using the ECST criteria, because both the residual lumen and the original diameter of the internal carotid artery can be evaluated at the specimen. The determination of the distal degree of stenosis at the specimen can only be measured with the help of the evaluation of the intraoperatively measured outside diameter of the distal "healthy" internal carotid with a micrometer. The consideration of the wall thickness, of 1 mm for all carotid arteries seems to be appropriate, but represents a small weakness of the methodology, although the difference between the local and distal degree of stenosis of about 4 – 7 % nearly corresponds to the known (and confirmed) difference between the ECST and NASCET data of about 8 – 10 %. As we see it, the quantification of the internal carotid stenosis at the specimen after conventional longitudinal arteriotomy is seldom possible. This is underlined by the small case number and the reported problems in methodology.

ad 2

Our results show that high-grade internal carotid stenoses will angiographically be underestimated up to 20 %. In particular, this refers to the aortic arch angiography, which results in a significant underestimation of the local and distal linear degree of stenosis. The sole aortic arch angiography is not suitable to reliably determine the degree of stenosis with a sensitivity of 85.2 % for the local degree of stenosis and only 60 % for the distal degree of stenosis of > 70 % stenoses. Partially, high-grade carotid stenoses will also clearly be underestimated by selective angiography, whereas moderate internal carotid stenoses (60 – 80 %) will be slightly overestimated as a tendency. The results of other authors were confirmed: Pan et al. reported in their study about 31 carotid specimen evaluated with MR angiography an angiographic underestimation of the stenoses in > 37 %, a conformity in 57 %, and an underestimation in 6 % (categories: 40 – 59 %, 60 – 79 %, 80 – 99 %, ECST criteria). They favored MR angiography and Duplex ultrasound, which both correctly classified the stenoses in 76 % and 75 % respectively (21). Our planimetric investigations showed that the planar degree of stenosis is higher as the linear degree of stenosis in 4 – 12 % (median) and the larger differences will be found in the group with the general angiography. Alexandrov et al. found out in their study of 15 planimetrically evaluated carotid specimens after conventional endarterectomy using the ECST criteria an angiographic underestimation of the stenoses of 13 % on average, and even of 19 % using the NASCET criteria. Duplex ultrasound was considered more valid in this study (1). CP Warlow and HJM Barnett, organizers of the ECST and the NASCET trials, point out that the superiority of carotid endarterectomy was proven in these studies mentioned above with angiographically quantified carotid stenoses (2). Besides that, it will not be allowed to compare the angiography as a 2-D technique to the planimetrically calculated planar degrees of stenosis. The discussion about an adequate diagnostic method prior to carotid endarterectomy will be aggravated by the fact that there are no larger studies validating Duplex and/or MR angiography with the help of the carotid specimen. As we see it, the systematic investigation of carotid eversion cylinders is able to overcome this deficiency, in order to precisely narrow the indication for the preoperative carotid angiography to special cases. The present criteria for the quantification and qualification (ulcer, stable-instable plaque) of carotid stenoses are not suitable to generally renounce the selective angiography for higher-grade carotid stenoses, except in rare cases (17, 22).

Conclusions

1) The planimetric investigation of carotid eversion cylinders provide the basis for the evaluation of the linear and planar degree of carotid stenosis directly at the site of the eversion endarterectomy (local degree of stenosis).

2) Extracranial high-grade carotid stenosis might easily be angiographically underestimated. A reliable quantification of > 70 % internal carotid artery stenosis is only possible with selective angiography. The aortic arch angiography significantly underestimates > 70 % carotid stenoses.

3) The planimetric investigation of carotid eversion cylinders appears to be appropriate to further evaluate other more or less invasive diagnostic techniques (Duplex, CT-, MR-angiography) in order to work out reliable criteria for the quantification of carotid stenoses.

References

1. Alexandrov AV, Bladdin CF, Maggisano R, Norris JW (1993) Measuring carotid Stenosis, time for a reappraisal. Stroke 24: 1292
2. Barnett HJM, Warlow CP (1993) Carotid endarterectomy and the measurement of stenosis. Stroke 24: 1281
3. Bladin CF, Alexandrov AV, Norris JW (1994) How should we measure carotid stenosis? The Lancet 344: 69
4. Blatter DD, Bahr AL, Parker DL, Robinson RO, Kimball JA, Perry DM, Horn S (1993) Cervical carotid MR Angiography with multiple overlapping thin-slab acquisition: comparison with conventional angiography. AJR 161: 1269
5. Dillon EH, van Leeuwen MS, Fernandez MA, Eikelboom BC, Mali WP (1993) CT angiography: application to the evaluation of carotid artery stenosis. Radiology 189: 211
6. v. Eckmann A, Schmiedt W, Störkel S, Kuhn FP (1990) Zur Diagnostik atherosklerotischer Läsionen der extrakraniellen Arteria carotis mit Duplex-Sonographie und IA-DSA, RoFo 153: 48

7. Eckstein HH, Post K, Hupp T, Weber F, Allenberg JR (1995) Die CT-Angiographie (CTA) von Carotisstenosen-Bestimmung des Stenosegrades im Vergleich zur konventionellen Angiographie. Zentralbl Chir, 120 (Suppl I): 40

8. Eckstein HH, Post K, Hoffmann E, Hupp T, Allenberg JR (1995) Bestimmung des Stenosegrades der A. carotis interna am Operationspräparat nach Eversions-TEA: Vergleich mit Angiographie und c-w-Doppler-Sonographie: VASA 24: 176

9. Etheredge SN (1970) A simple technique for carotid endarterectomy. Ann Surg 120: 275

10. European Carotid Surgery Trialist's Collaborative Group (1991) MRC European carotid surgery trial: interim results for symptomatic patients with severe (70 – 99 %) or with mild (0 – 29 %) carotid stenosis. Lancet 337: 1235

11. Fischer GG, Anderson DC, Farber R, Lebow S (1985) Prediction of carotid disease by ultrasound and digital subtraction angiography. Arch Neurol 42: 224

12. Fox AJ (1993) How to measure carotid stenosis. Radiology 186: 316

13. Fox CH, Johnson FB, Whiting J, Roller PP (1985) Formaldehyde fixation. J Histochem Cytochem 33: 845

14. Hobson RW, Strandness DE (1993) Carotid artery stenosis: what's in the measurement? J Vasc Surg 18: 1069

15. Hupp T, Eckstein HH, Frankenberg M, Schaible A, Allenberg JR (1994) Verfahrenswechsel zur Eversions-TEA der Arteria carotis interna: Erfahrungen bei den ersten 300 Operationen. Zentralbl Chir 119 (Suppl): 90

16. Marks MP, Napel S, Jordan JE, Enzmann DR (1993) Diagnosis of carotid artery disease: preliminary experience with maximum-intensity-projection spiral CT angiography. Am J Roentgenol 160: 1276

17. Masryk TJ, Obuchowski NA (1993) Noninvasive carotid imaging: caveat emptor. Radiology 186: 325

18. Moneta GL, Edwards JM, Chitwood RW, Taylor LM, Lee RW, Cummings CA, Porter JM (1993) Correlation of North American Symptomatic Endarterectomy trial (NASCET) angiographic definition of 70 % to 99 % internal carotid artery stenosis with duplex scanning. J Vasc Surg 17: 152

19. Norris JW, Chucz ZU, Bernstein NM, Chambers BR (1991) Vascular risks of asymptomatic carotid stenosis. Stroke 22: 1485

20. North American Symptomatic Carotid Endarterectomy Trial Collaborators (1991): benefical effect of carotid endarterectomy in symptomatic patients with high-grade carotid stenosis. N Engl J Med 1325: 445

21. Pan XM, Saloner D, Reilly LM, Bowersox JC, Murray SP, Anderson CM, Gooding GAW, Rapp JH (1995) Assessment of carotid artery stenosis by ultrasonography, conventional angiography and magnetic resonance angiography: correlation with ex vivo measurement of plaque stenosis. J Vasc Surg 21: 82

22. Polak JF (1993) Noninvasive carotid evaluation: carpe diem. Radiology 186: 329

23. Ricotta JJ, Bryan FA, Bond MC, Kurtz A, O'Leary DH, Raines JK, Berson AS, Clouse ME, Calderson-Oritz M, Toole JF, De Weese JA, Smullens SN, Gustafson NF (1987) Validation of real time ultrasound, arteriography and pathology. Sensitivity and specifity. J Vasc Surg 6: 512

24. Rothwell PM, Gibson RJ, Slattery J, Sellar RJ, Warlow CP for the European Carotid Surgery Trialists' Collaborative Group (1994) Equivalence of measurements of three methods on 1001 angiograms. Stroke 25: 2435

25. Schenk EA, Bond GM, Aretz TH, Angelo JN, Choi HY, Rynalski TR, Gustafson NF, Berson AS, Ricotta JJ, Goodison MW, Bryan FA, Goldberg BB, Toole JF, O'Leary DH (1988) Multicenter validation study of real-time ultrasonography, arteriography and pathology: pathologic evaluation of carotid endarterectomy specimens. Stroke 19: 289

26. Schwartz RB, Jones JM, Chernoff DM, Mukherji SK, Khorasani R, Tice HM, Kikinis R, Hooton SM, Szieg PE, Polak JF (1992) Common carotid artery bifurcation: evaluation with spiral CT-work in progress. Radiology 185: 513

27. Sheldon JJ, Janowitz W, Leborgne JM, Silvina M, Rojo N (1984) Intravenous DSA of extracranial carotid lesions: comparison with other techniques and specimens. Am J Reontgenol 143: 1289

28. Spencer MP, Reid JM (1979) Quantitation of carotid stenosis with continuous-wave (c-w) Doppler ultrasound. Stroke 10: 326

29. Widder B, Friedrich JM, Paulat K, Hamann H, Hutschenreiter S, Kreutzer C, Ott F, Arlart IP (1987) Bestimmung des Stenosierungsgrades bei Karotisstenosen: Ultraschall und i.v. DSA im Vergleich zum Operationsbefund. Ultraschall 8: 82

30. Williams MA, Nicolaidis AN (1987) Predicting the normal dimensions of the internal and external carotid arteries from the diameter of the common carotid. Eur J Vasc Surg 1: 91

Author's address:
Dr. H.-H. Eckstein
Department of Surgery
Division of Vascular Surgery
Im Neuenheimer Feld 110
69120 Heidelberg, Germany

Consensus conference on perioperative monitoring

W. S. Moore

I am struck with a couple of observations that have come my way while listening to the talks of this really excellent meeting, and I thought it might be helpful just to give a little bit of a perspective overview before we attempt to address the questions that Dr. Horsch has asked us to do.

I think that to begin with I would like to just state the obvious in that the objective of monitoring (I use the term in the broader sense – that is both the anatomic and the physiologic) really is to reduce the incidence of postoperative neurologic morbidity and mortality.

The problem that we run into is that there are at least two major categories that can result in a postoperative neurological deficit. One has to do with the damage that is done during the period of carotid artery cross-clamping, which is where most of our physiologic testing that is done today is directed. The second has to to with the technical problems that can occur as a consequence of some misadventure during the procedure itself. The problem is that the endpoint of both of those is exactly the same and to be able to separate what caused one versus the other is very difficult. Those who have addressed the ratio between technical problems causing postoperative deficit versus intraoperative clamping resulting in postoperative deficit suggest that by far the majority of these are technical causes and not clamping. Even in Dr. Ackerstaff's presentation today he showed at least 2/3rds of those that they identified were technical and 1/3rd were related to the clamp-procedure itself. And so I would suggest that perhaps at least as much effort be directed towards improving technical result as it is at detecting difficulties associated with clamping. In a recent study in which we attempted to identify surgeons who were technically competent to participate in a trial – specifically the 'Eyckhouse' study – one of the things that became evident was: Should we, or should we not try to standardize the surgical procedure including monitoring? It became evident very quickly that we would never be able to do that because each surgeon had his own concept of technique: Patch versus no patch; shunt versus no shunt; and so forth. Certainly they all had their own concept of what would be the best way of monitoring the patient, whether it be back pressure, electroencephalography (EEG), somatosensory evoked potential (SEP), transcranial doppler (TCD); combinations of the above – and so what we decided to do was to settle with what we call the "bottom line": Is the result satisfactory? Is the complication rate in the individual surgeon's hands sufficiently low to justify their doing or participating in the trial?

I think that we will come up with the following today: If we define consensus as a general agreement, we will certainly not reach this with regard to an approach or in terms of an individual procedure. What we may, thus, be able to do is to agree to the fact that we are going to disagree on the very best method for each of the procedures that we have talked about. Does that mean we should start looking? – Certainly not! But I would suggest that whatever works best in an individual's hands is what ought to be used!

S. Horsch

Thank you very much, Dr. Moore!

Well, Ladies and Gentlemen, the principal aim of this meeting was to state what monitoring methods we have access to and experience with, and the aim of the congress should be – can we give a recommendation to all the other vascular surgeons – should they apply intraoperative monitoring control or not, should they shunt or not – and this under the aspect of quality control that is performed in principal today, but we have to justify legally tomorrow. For this reason we prepared six points for discussion. All the specialists here were involved and are present to discuss and state their opinion as to how they feel about these recommendations.

I would like to start with point number 1: A basic definition and the necessity of perioperative monitoring, and when we focus on point 1a, the anaesthesiological monitoring.

I apologize Dr. Abel for picking on you to open the discussion round, but to my knowledge you are the only anaesthetist present at this the table. What is your opinion?

M. Abel

As already presented this morning during my lecture, I feel that, first of all, prior to induction of general anaesthesia we should consider the general risk profile of each individual patient. Therefore, in my opinion monitoring should entail primarily the monitoring of intraarterial blood pressure, secondly an electrocardiogram, thirdly pulse oxymetry, and if the procedure is performed under general anaesthesia, one should also monitor the capnometry.

All others should be discussed later in this session with the questions focusing on the intraoperative cerebral monitoring. But I as an anaesthesiologist would say that these four parameters are always in need of monitoring, irrespective of other aspects.

S. Horsch

Thank you; are the panellists in agreement with this?

G. Hagmüller

I agree completely with this because I think every kind of intraoperative monitoring that we have developed is absolutely necessary for us to be aware of the fine margins of our complication rates. We have seemingly convinced most neurologists that carotid endarterectomy in specific cases is superior to conservative treatment – and if we don't further decrease our currently low percentage of complications down to a near zero level, neurologists may hesitate, in fact they may even change their minds about referrals should the complication rate rise correspondingly with the carotid endarterectomy now becoming a procedure which is performed by an increasing number of vascular surgeons with possibly less experience. Therefore, accurate monitoring as a means of quality control is absolutely necessary.

M. Abel

I would like to add some more to the discussion as to whether we should do the procedure under general anaesthesia or locoregional anaesthesia; I do not think this is the crux of the matter. In modern anaesthesia the complication rate is close to zero. I think you should first of all look at your patient and at the risk profile of your patient. And if an anaesthesia, which is able to take pain as well as sympathetic overdrive, is also able to reduce the genuine risk profile of your patient, then you should opt for this procedure or this particular technique. In my opinion, general anaesthesia in experienced hands is as safe as close to zero percent complications as incured by the method. Further, it is able to reduce the individual patient's risks at a cardiovascular level, a respiratory level, a metabolic level, as well as the level of renal insufficiency. For these reasons I think the discussion should not center around whether to use ancient techniques from ancient times, but we should focus our attention on our present day patients. These patients are daily coming to be of a more advanced age with a concurrent rise in morbidity, and so we are forced to focus on this new patient. And in these times I think we should monitor as much as possible if we want to reduce a complication rate to 1 per 3 %. It will be much more costly and require more expertise and intelligence than to have reduced a complication rate from five or eight points as in former times.

A. Imparato

At the risk of not making sense, I would like to state two facts: Firstly, there is only one technique of monitoring that has been successful for 35 years; that is monitoring of the conscious patient. It has never had to go through a period where the stroke rate was 35 % as it was in trying to work out whether the carotid stump pressure was of any value. It has never had to go through a period where people had to learn something that was already known, and that is that the electroencephalogram monitors the surface of the brain; it does not monitor to the deep portions of the brain; patients have actually died with electroencephalograms that looked normal and so on and so forth with every other monitoring technique except local anaesthesia. That is fact number one.

Fact number two: There has been only one protective technique that has protected the brain from ischaemia or has reversed it and that is the shunt. We tried CO_2 inhalations, we tried Diamox, we tried artificial hypertension, and so on and so forth. General anaesthesia has been tried, and it is only the shunt that has reversed an ischaemic brain to a non-ischaemic brain. Artificial hypertension is too dangerous to use. So here we have two facts: 1. – monitoring the conscious patient is effective and it has never failed; 2. – the shunt is a proven way of reversing cerebral ischaemia.

The only problem with the shunt is that it gets in the way of doing a difficult operation and it can be a pathway for embolization. This is the reason why I think monitoring needs to be done.

Now, the 3rd fact is that I believe my group was the first group to publish an analysis of the specific courses of postoperative or intraoperative neurological deficits. It was possible to do this because we were doing the procedure with our patients awake, and we could very clearly differentiate between intraoperative embolization in clamping ischaemia – if the patient suffers clamping ischaemia on the operating table, then you remove the clamp and the patient recovers almost immediately. If the patient is embolised, then the defect presists for a while. And so we know that the incidence of clamping ischaemia in a well-run series is about 0.5 %. The conclusion of our work was that the majority of the neurologic deficits that occurred were due to technical errors with one exeption and that is: we did not know the cause of intracerebral haemorrhage, whose incidence by the way has decreased. As far as I can say. there is no problem. You monitor the patient awake, you always get the right answer, and if the patient will not tolerate what you are doing, you put in a shunt. A shunt is put in a certain way and I don't see what all the other complexity is about, or why it is necessary. This is an arguement that has been going on for 35 years, since I was a boy, and I'm not a boy anymore. So, I would love it if somebody could enlighten me on why we have to go through this – is it the built careers, is it the right papers, it is certainly not to help patients, because they can be helped in other ways.

I learned a very important lesson from Dr. C. Walton Lillehei if I may: In the early days of open-heart surgery, we had terrible difficulties getting our patients to survive the pump-run. So I was sent out to C Walton Lillehei, who had the most magnificent record of fixing hearts. He took the simplest and yet most complex and laborious system for perfusing a heart. What he was interested in doing was fixing the heart, not learning how to perfuse it more efficiently; he had an efficient method. He kept the patients alive; he could do the procedure while the rest of us were struggling trying to figure out whether to use bubble-oxygenators. I think we are in the same situation with carotids, except we are 35 years later. He learned it in a year or two. We have not learned it as vascular surgeons for 35 years. Could somebody enlighten me?

P. Fiorani

There is a fact about the local anaesthesia and that is it needs to be performed efficiently by the colleague, the anaesthesiologist. Yet we are the ones who perform the operation. The involvement of the anaesthesiologist may, therefore, be a bit more than usual because he has the complete control of the neurological condition of the patient. Coming to the point of the anaesthesiological monitoring, it was never proven that we are operating in local anaesthesia with the same kind of monitoring. Coming back to what Dr. Imperato said, when we moved to the first steps in the carotid endarterectomy, we believed that the first point to ensure was the monitoring of cerebral circulation. We worked many, many years ago in the 60's/65's in cooperation with Dr. Larsen, Copenhagen, and we also published an editorial in 1971 and then also performed experiments with the best system of monitoring of cerebral circulation, that is with Technetium clearance. This was then the gold standard for three years. Then we compared this gold standard (the Xenon Clearance Study) with all the others such as stump pressure, etc, and evaluated this metal and then started to operate using a much simpler intra-operative monitoring technique, the EEG. But we noticed numerous mistakes and even when applying the best available monitor, we always have a certain rate of neurological complications that could not be explained on the basis of our at that time considered excellent monitoring system. For this reason it may be that the competitor will go to local anaesthesia. Because we believe our surgical complication rate to be low with a morbidity and mortality of 1.5 % to 2 %, we cannot run the risk that this rate rises to over 1 % due to a wrong system of monitoring. The point is, if I see the excellent presentations from today in which one system of monitoring has supposedly a sensitivity of 98 %, which is undoubtedly very high, the suitability still remains questionable to me, when the patient is left with a total mortality risk of between 1.5 and 2 %. This is the reason why we, following Dr. Imparato, moved our monitoring to the form using local anaesthesia.

B. Habozit

I agree completely with Dr. Imperato and Dr. Fiorani. Five years ago in France only 10 % of anaesthesias were locoregional, and in 1995 52 % of anaesthesias were locoregional. I think in this way neurological monotoring is excellent with a 100 % sensitivity and anaesthesiologists need to make the best possible situation out of this kind of anaesthesia.

M. Abel

Dr. Imperato, I would like to make the following differentiation: In my opinion, the starting point for the surgical intervention is very important. If you are faced with a wake patient who is running into the risk of developing a sympathetic overdrive situation and is additionally a multimorbid patient from a cardiovascular point of view, etc., then this is a double bladed sword. Our aim to attain an optimally stable patient prior to surgical intervention is on one side. This to me is one of the indications for general anaesthesia in order to stabilize the vital functions. The second side to the story is the monitoring; I agree completely with you that a wake patient provides a very good and simple monitoring. All the sophisticated techniques available for monitoring the anaesthetized patient during carotid surgery are certainly in no way superior to the wake patient. I, therefore, agree with you completely on the statement that the wake patient is the finest available form of monitoring, but the indication for a general anaesthesia is not only dependent on the cerebral monitoring, but in the first line to provide a stable surrounding intra- and extracorporally, to stabilize homeostasis, and to prevent the development of secondary risks on cardiac functions.

A. Imperato

With all due respects to the anaesthesia community, general anaesthesia is not a stable state. It is probably as dramatically taxing to a patient as any technique can ever be. I can also tell you that for years I used to be accused of trying to kill my patients by operating on them while they were awake. What they said was 'you are taking these patients with coronary artery disease, you subject them to stress, and you are giving them heart attacks.' That turned out not to be true; as a matter of fact our conviction is that the reverse is probably true! Finally, I mention a fact that is not totally explained, but I think it to be very important. It came out of the Veterans Administration Study for which I was on the data monitoring committee. It is very impressive and wasn't thought about for a long time that those patients who are subjected to the general anaesthesia and have their carotids fixed had a higher late myocardial infarction rate than the patients who were medically treated. Now I don't know what the explanation of that is, but that fits in with something that I had noticed as a clinician. If a certain number of patients have general anaesthesia, they have a heart-attack because there are these massive fluid shifts that can occur. There is all kinds of stuff that the body has to do which is stressful, so I don't consider general anaesthesia either non-stressful or a stable state.

I think this is such an important issue. I do not think I have the data to prove it, nor do you. I remember the day when it used to be said that you put the patients to sleep so as to protect the brain, and we went through all our discussion with no proof. So, I don't think we have anymore proof that general anaesthesia is more effective than local, except the minuscule difference that we have been able to show. And I think it is such a critical issue, especially since patients are having both their hearts fixed and their brains revascularized, that the way in which it should be done to get the maximum retrieval is not established and it is worthwhile to have a rigidly controlled, prospective randomized clinical trial.

W. S. Moore

As a surgeon I'd like to take just a moment to defend general anaesthesia for carotid endadorectomy and I think all of the points that Dr. Imparato made are absolutely correct with respect to intraoperative monitoring of the awake patient. Having gone through an experience both in local anaesthesia or surgical block anaesthesia, in general anaesthesia I can tell you from a personal perspective that there is no way that I wish to go back to local anaesthesia. That has nothing to do with the patients, it has to do with me and how well I do the operation. If you are working in an unusual anatomic circumstance, if you have a very high carotid bifurcation or if you have a high lesion then you have to get up and start working in the area at the base of the skull. I have not yet seen a surgical block anaesthetic that will make the patient comfortable during that period of time and inevitably what starts to happen is that the patient becomes somewhat uncomfortable, begins to move, and for this particular reason I become uncomfortable. I think I would in this situation not perform as good an operation as I will wish the patient totally asleep, not agitated and not moving, and so when you have a patient who gets very uncomfortable, begins to move, twist and turn, you need more than a cool surgeon, you need a surgeon, who has a temperature somewhere between cool and absolute zero and this surgeon I have yet to meet. In summary, I need general anaesthesia in order to do a good job.

A. Imparato

Well, I would take another point of view; I don't consider the patient population to be my oyster. I concider myself to be the servant to the patient. If I cannot do something properly in the best interest of the patient, then I don't do it! Point number one that is what medicine is all about!

Secondly when surgeons talk about being at the the base of the skull and not at the base of the skull, they're just fitting a styloid process. One has about another mile and a half to go before reaching the base of the skull. If one will simply learn to break the styloid process that block will do fine, you'll get up as high as you need to, and we do it! The point is, we do it! It is not something that is mentioned on a theoretical basis; you cannot argue with the fact that it has been done, and it has been done successfully – we have not had to go through a whole lot of 33 % stroke rate in order to prove that something is not good. This is good; it works.

H. M. Becker

As far as anaesthesiological monitoring is concerned, we are surgeons; we all agree with what Dr. Abel said in that it is very important to have a continuous arterial pressure monitoring and ECG monitoring maybe also the pulse oxymetry, and I would like to add – a urinary catheter. This is not that important intraoperatively but ever so more postoperatively.

But concerning the intraoperative cerebral monitoring I think we have to differentiate between two kinds of ischaemias. I learned from Dr. DeBakey that a postoperative neurological deficit is a surgical failure, a technical failure of the surgeon, because of intraoperative embolisation during preparation or anything else. It is really a technical failure and I think Dr. Ackerstaff was the first today who differentiated between these two different kinds of ischaemias: the embolisation or original ischaemia and the global ischaemia.

Concerning global ischaemia, I am not convinced that monitoring such as SEP or transcranial Oxymetry is necessary, although I do most certainly consider them both fit for detecting global ischaemia of the brain induced by cross-clamping. When we see that many centers never use a shunt as for example Dr. Dzsinich in Budapest; he would never use a shunt. Am I correct with my statement?

C. Dzsinich

Not never, but definitely only rather occasionally.

H. M. Becker

Dr. Raithel also does not principally use intra-operative shunting.

S. Horsch

May I point out here that Dr. Raithel is using intra-operative monitoring, even though this does not have the use of a shunt as a consequence.

H. M. Becker

Principally never using a shunt and performing up to 1000 procedures per year that is the standard of Dr. Raithel. I would like to bring up the point of using routine shunting and thereby avoiding laborious monitoring methods. We have adopted this approach for our carotid endarterectomies: all our patients are routinely shunted. In my opinion the detection of cerebral embolisation is only possible using the transcranial doppler for monitoring or by an intraoperative angiography. We have had a lot of positive experience using the intra-operative angiography, and I would like to promote this as a vital procedure in order to detect an embolic occlusion of the middle cerebral artery (MCA). If this is timely detected, a local thrombolysis of this embolization may be attempted. Therefore, in my eyes nobody should abstain from the intra-operative angiography where it is possible to perform such.

S. Horsch

Refering back to the first point, I think we all agree that anaesthesiological monotoring is vital and we should not ponder over the question of whether to use local or general anaesthesia any longer, or else we will have missed the point. We are here to discuss the necessity of surgical monitoring.

Progressing on to intraoperative cerebral monitoring, we heard this morning about all the methods available to us; and shunting should also be included as a monitoring method here, but this a method that necessitates supervision. Getting back to all the methods we heard about: Stump pressure, EEG, SEP, TCD, Oxymetry and other methods. I would be interested in your individual opinions to these. What is your range used; what is your personal recommendation to the auditorium? What would you place at first priority, at number two?

Dr. Becker, you told us you do not require any of the mentioned methods, you will always shunt.

H. M. Becker

Correct – I follow DeBakey's 3 's' rule: simple, safe, short.

S. Horsch

SEP would succumb to this; it is simple, safe and short. Shunt is simple, short, but can be dangerous.

H. M. Becker

Yes, but all these things have to be practical and it has to be inexpensive. You require competent and well-trained personnel for accurate SEP monitoring. We have equivalently good results as you do, so I do not see any need to further elaborate on my monitoring devices with SEP or a transcranial Oxymetry. It sure has a scientific aspect, but I am not convinced of its clinical relevance for the practice of carotid surgery.

S. Horsch

You seem to be the more competent shunter of the two of us. It would interest me to hear the opinion of Dr. Dzsinich. What is your indication for shunting?

C. Dzsinich

As I have already told you; we seldomly use a shunt. Our young colleagues went to Dr. Raithel in Nuremberg for further training and returned only to convert our previous surgical technique of carotid endarterectomy into an eversion technique, which we are extremely satisfied with. We used the shunt in the early years of carotid surgery, seldom in the early 90s and hardly ever these days. If we are confronted with any difficulties, we apply an interposition graft, but shunting is used extremely rarely at our clinic at present.

S. Horsch

Thank you, Dr. Dzsinich. Dr. Balzer, what is your opinion?

K. Balzer

If we are performing a carotid endarterectomy, this can be classified as an operation of the brain. For this reason, we should use a monitoring method which provides us with an indication of what is happening in the brain. The SEP is the only method available which gives us this information directly and in the most reliant manner, and it is an easy to apply method. Furthermore, it is inexpensive, and in my opinion it also gives us a clear indication of when to put in a shunt. In summary, I, therefore, consider evoked potentials as the best presently available method for intraoperative control.

S. Horsch

So in your opinion the monitoring of choice is SEP?

K. Balzer

That is correct.

S. Horsch

Dr. Eckstein, may we hear what the situation is in Heidelberg?

H. H. Eckstein

Our first choice is also SEP, but I would like to point out that after listening to the presentations today, our results seem so perfect; there almost seems to be no room for improvements. We registered a complication rate of only 1 % or less and the question arises of how necessary the monitoring really is?

But if you look at the results of the NASCET study, the ECST study, or other studies, the complication rate was much higher previously, up to 7.5 %. I guess that this is reality maybe not for us at present but for the whole society of vascular surgery, and those colleagues, as well as trainees in vascular surgery, need a monitoring system that gives one time and the security and safety to do a perfect endarterectomy. Therefore, we always need SEP, as well as a completion angiography in order to detected technical failures and thromboses. We strongly feel that we should then be able to lower our complication rates by up to 1 to 2 % by having used these additional methods.

S. Horsch

I agree with you that a 1 % complication rate is indeed very low. But please remember, we are increasingly operating on asymptomatic patients. If this patient falls into the 1 % range, then this is 1 % too much.

R. G. A. Ackerstaff

That is also reinforcing my comment. When you work in an institution where you can rely on the data and on the assessment and analysis of the data and you have a perioperative stroke rate of 1 % or less, then of course this is very hard to decrease, no matter how many modalities of intraoperative monitoring are applied. We have to realize, however, that we are talking about the best numerical results here. Somewhere there must be an enormous bias in publication of success rates of carotid surgery, for we all know that there are centers where the morbidity and mortality rate is much higher. And the very moment we realize that in the near future we will operate more and more on asymptomatic patients, I would not like to be the patient who had an asymptomatic stenosis and awake with a minor stroke of my left hemisphere.

So, I think we will reach the point even in Europe where the law will demand from us that we monitor all patients and that we have to do this in the safest possible way. And in my personal view, if you have reached the conclusion to perform intraoperative monitoring of brain function, I would opt for a combination of EEG and SEP. It needs to be computerized in order to provide the surgeon with clear-cut evidence for the necessity of implanting a shunt, and not be labeled as a 'possibly slight decrease' in EEG activity or 'latency in SEP by 25 or 26 %'. The indication needs to be given a numerical form, which must be computerized and standardized of course, and the TCD does provide a helpful additional criterium indicating the flow in the feeding artery of the brain volume for completeness sake. Roughly 300 to 500 g is dependent on the perfusion via the MCA during cross-clamping.

I consider the advantages of the TCD over the other two modalities enormous when one assesses them in terms of haemodynamic insides, but also of course in terms of the insides of embolisation, what impact embolisation has, and how meticolous the surgical procedure was performed. Also in our institution many surgeons who have performed carotid surgery for more than 10 years thought that their flushing was correctly done. The very moment they had a TCD, they realized that flushing can also introduce microemboli, via external and periobiteral arteries, and into the ipsilateral MCA. Even at their stage of surely great experience, there was sometimes a significant embolisation noticed during clamp release. TCD, thus, provides one with enormous insight into all these pathophysiologic mechanisms as well as supplying immediate feed-back to the surgeon on his accuracy while operating on that particular patient and may help him improve the next procedure.

S. Horsch

Well, Dr. Ackerstaff, combined EEG and SEP monitoring may be too complex and too difficult for most institutions. What is your first choice of these two?

R. G. A. Ackerstaff

I meant that only one of these should be applied, not both simultaneously. I am not quite sure which of these two I would give preference to. I do not think that we have enough information available to decide on either one or the other at this stage. As far as I know, there are no publications with large numbers which have been able to prove the superiority of one over the other. I have thought about it in theory and have a tendency to personally opt for the EEG in theoretical terms, but I have no scientific justification for this. To me the SEP does not really make sense, I consider it a varification of the EEG monitoring.

S. Horsch

Dr. Loeprecht, what do you think? Do you need monitoring or not?

H. Loeprecht

Of course I am convinced that we need some sort of monitoring, especially considering that the patient is under general anaesthesia and he cannot demonstrate his motor activity, etc. Therefore, we need a system of monitoring, and we start by using the EEG. The problem is that in order to be convinced of the effectiveness of a method, one must have extracted numerous neurological deficits and this means that in total one has to collect a massive number of EEG records in order to find these deficits. This was precisely the problem with our study: In the patient group of 150, there were 5 neurological events. A single one not detected by the EEG reduced its sensitivity noteably. In my opinion it would be worthwhile to start a large study for either the SEP or the EEG in a multi-center project in order to detect the true effectiveness by assessing a thousand or so cases.

S. Horsch

But currently you have no special favor for SEP or EEG?

H. Loeprecht

No, we have only used the EEG. It is an accurate recording; one has a precise documentation during the course of the operation. We do not rely on it for selecting the patient necessitating a shunt, but use it for accurate documentation of the whole concept.

S. Horsch

Dr. Sciacca, what is your opinion?

V. Sciacca

I consider the idea of local anaesthesia not feasible for many reasons, including the anxiety of the patient. We use EEG monitoring with 32 leads as we have no TCD or SEP available, but I think that the SEP is probably more sensitive than the EEG in clarifiying what is going on deep in the brain.

S. Horsch

Well, I think I can summarize up to this point by saying that we generally all agree that we need intraoperative monitoring varying between the different institutions in the form of either SEP or EEG.

A. Imparato

I would like to make a comment here. Dr. Jesse Thompson probably has as much experience as anybody in the world will ever have, and he still is an advocate of routine shunting.

So whichever side one picks one comes to this point again.

S. Horsch

Agreed upon, but let us refrain from discussing whether or not to shunt, or else we will still be at this tomorrow.

A special point in this intraoperative monitoring question is the quality control. I think we are in particular need of the since introduction of the new technique, the eversion technique. We now need to critically look at what we have desobliterated. We discussed earlier today the intaoperative angioscopy and angiography. Dr.

Balzer, I would be interested in your opinion on this. Do we need a quality control in the form of angiography or angioscopy with the new eversion technique?

K. Balzer

I am sure we need at least one of these techniques as a routine method. When doing an eversion endarterectomy, it should be sufficient in most cases to do an angioscopic control following the endarterectomy. If this is satisfying, then the operation may be completed. In cases of doubt, an angiogram should be performed after completion of the operation. In the literature a complication rate of 6 to 10 % following inadequately performed control angiograms is documented, and for this reason I emphasize that a careful selection of patients requiring an angiogram should be practised. It is most certainly not necessary to perform this routinely.

H. H. Eckstein

We also prefer on-table angiography, but have no experience with angioscopy. It may very well suffice to perform the angioscopy, but the angiography additionally provides one with the opportunity of demonstrating the intracranial arteries in cases where an SEP loss over 3 to 5 minutes occurred, but it was decided not to shunt. All of us know this situation where we are not quite sure, and we then perform the angiography of the carotid bifurcation and the intracranial vessels. In this way we ensure that the main stem of the middle cerebral artery and the anterior cerebral artery is patent. A postoperative control angiogram in cases of neurological deficits, thus, becomes superfluous, and we can be relatively sure that these deficits are of the TIA form.

S. Horsch

Can we agree then that when using the conventional desobliteration technique or when the entire operation field is visualized, we in all these cases do not need a quality control. However, when using the new eversion technique, we then do require a control in order to assess what we have done?

W. S. Moore

I do not think, I would agree on that point. It is somewhere between 66 and 99 % of the postoperative complications that are technical. I think we have to be absolutely certain that we are leaving the operating table with the best possible technical result. From my perspective there are 3 ways in doing that; two of which have been discussed: the completion angiography and the angioscopy. The third is the possibility of using Duplex scanning on the operating table. But I think that one of those three imaging methods is mandatory. In my hands the best thing is a completion angiogram because that not only gives me information about the operative field, but also about the intracranial circulation.

If we are willing to do completion angiograms when we do a tibial bypass when the worst thing that can happen is a thrombosed graft and a trip back to the operating room at night, then why should we not do an angiogram when the complication is a non-reversible stroke?

S Horsch

This is a very good point, and I think we are now all convinced that we need intraoperative monitoring and that we need quality control when using the eversion technique.

Now coming to the third point: the intensive care unit (ICU). I would first of all like to ask those colleagues performing the procedure under local anaesthesia: what monitoring do you use postoperatively in the ICU for the patient who has been operated on under local anaesthesia?

A. Imparato

Blood pressure, respiration, and neurological status are very easy to monitor if they have been done under local anaesthesia. They are responsive, they have not been heavily sedated, pain is not a major problem – so they are very easy to monitor. The biggest problem is, as in any patient who has received an anticoagulant, the monitoring for the haematoma in the neck, which is rare but can occur. I think one must very carefully watch for that, so much so that one does not put any dressings on the neck or after a couple of hours just take the dressings off.

S. Horsch

I would like to pose another question to you. Do we really need to routinely transfer every patient after an endarterectomy to the ICU?

H. M. Becker

Usually the carotid patient is not an ICU patient. And I can only see one reason to refer the patient to the ICU: the hypertensive crisis. Otherwise, the patient needs one day of intermediate care and on the second day he can be released.

A. Imparato

I think the blood pressure is a critical issue. Our patients have hypotensive crises, not hypertensive crises. We ascribe it to the local procedure. We, many years ago, got tired of making holes in that little artery of the crotch. So, we began to save the baroreceptor apparatus. Dr. Moore does not agree with me, he thinks that the blood pressure response is central, at least that is what I read from what he has said. I feel that the hypertensive crisis may be in part related to the fact that the baroreceptor is destroyed. So I do no dissection virtually at the bifurcation itself and save those little nerves. Since then we have been having no more trouble with postoperative hypertension, we don't get hypertensive crises, whereas in the past I had seen them frequently.

S. Horsch

Thank you, and progressing to the patient who received general anaesthesia, Dr. Abel, what do you think?

M. Abel

I my opinion we should monitor blood pressure, respiration, diuresis, and the electrocardiogram over a four to six hour period postoperatively. This should suffice.

S. Horsch

But do you believe that this needs to be done in an ICU?

M. Abel

This should be a decision made postoperatively involving the surgeon as well as the other disciplines; it is not generally necessary.

H. Loeprecht

The patient is observed in the recovery room postoperatively for 6 hours at our institution and is then transferred to the ward. This is feasible thanks to the well-trained nursing staff available to us.

S. Horsch

Dr. Becker, what is your opinion?

H. M. Becker

As I have mentioned, for our patients we have intermediate care beds where there is ECG monitoring and a control of the fluid balance is performed for 24 hours. Following this, the patients go to the wards fully mobilized.

K. Balzer

We use the approach that they use in Augsburg. The patients are observed for about 6 hours in the recovery room and after that they go to the normal ward. Here, they are then obviously observed by the nurse, who continuously controls the blood pressure and neurological functions according to a standardized scheme.

P. Fiorani

Patients who received local anaesthesia are sent to the recovery room for 6 to 12 hours in order to monitor haemodynamic condition and to be able to pick up any neurological symptoms at the first onset of symptoms.

S. Horsch

So we all agree that ICU or Intermediate Care is necessary in order to control vital functions as well as the neurological status postoperatively. May I ask you, Dr. Moore, what is your opinion and would you with in a few words summarize what we have discussed.

W. S. Moore

What we are doing at the present time is a brief period of observation in the recovery room – maybe two or four hours. If the patient is stable, neurologically intact, and he has no need for intravenous blood pressure medication, they go directly to the ward. They do not require monitoring after that.

A. Imparato

I have a question. At what day postoperatively has the group seen acute myocardial infarctions? We have seen them as late as the third day, when the patient was on the way out of the hospital on his way home. I don't know the solution for that problem. Is there anything we should be doing to catch these acute myocardial infarcts that occur as late as the third day?

M. Abel

It is not surprising; it is the same problem we are faced with in the cardiac surgery unit where the maximum of complications occur on the third to fifth postoperative day. I do not wish to repeat our initial discussion, but not only me, also numerous cardiocirculatory physicians and physiologists are of the opinion that hyperadreanargic situations and also hyperadreanargic situations in the sense of compensatory reactions of the individual could be the reason for these poor outcomes. These are relatively seldom, yet very tragic individual situations, and I think this is one of the best reasons why we should attempt to minimize all sympathetic overdrive in the patient. This applies not only to during the operation as discussed, but also to the preoperative period and the early postoperative period. It is important that when you put the patient back into his surrounding, the vegetative overdrive inside of him is working at its maximum. One can only use this up to the level, where the compensatory mechanisms are able to counteract this force and result in a positive effect. If he falls into a noradrenergic overdrive, you are on the risky side of ending up with a cardiocirculatory complication.

A. Imparato

Can you do measure the intravascular catecholamine levels?

M. Abel

Yes. We have studied these levels in cardiac surgery at the pre-, intra- and postoperative stage, and you can document these sympathetic overdrive situations.

I do not think that these levels should be determined routinely, but only in individual situations. There is an early indicator test available, which is easily performed. It is called CKMB, a kind of creatinine kinase enzyme specific for the myocardial tissue, and within 4 to 6 hours after anything has gone wrong in the coronary circulation, you register an acute rise of this CKMB parameter.

W. S. Moore

I think one other item that is helpful in the prevention of perioperative myocardial infarction is the routine use of preoperative aspirin. I do not know if others are doing that, but we keep them on aspirin right up to the time of surgery, as well as continuing to administer it postoperatively. It has been well documented that aspirin is a far better drug in preventing myocardial infarction than it is in preventing stroke.

S. Horsch

Well, Ladies and Gentlemen, we should end here as time has advanced on us. I think we all had a very interesting and rewarding day.

I would like to extend a special thanks to the panelists for presenting us with such a stimulating discussion.